CURRENT TRENDS IN THE MANAGEMENT OF BREAST CANCER

CURRENT TRENDS in the MANAGEMENT of BREAST CANCER

Edited by

R. ROBINSON BAKER, M.D.

Professor of Surgery and Oncology
The Johns Hopkins University School
of Medicine

The Johns Hopkins University Press

Baltimore and London

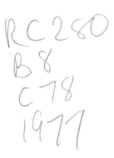

The Johns Hopkins University Press, Baltimore, Maryland 21218
The Johns Hopkins Press Ltd., London

Library of Congress Catalog Card Number 76-49094
ISBN 0-8018-1858-3

Library of Congress Cataloging in Publication data will be found on the last printed
page of this book.

To Jean Harvey Baker

CONTENTS

PREFACE

In this book we have attempted to present and correlate the recent literature on carcinoma of the breast, particularly as it relates to clinical practice. The book is not a complete or definitive text on the subject. It does present the clinician with a review of the current literature on the epidemiology, pathology, radiology, and clinical management of breast cancer. The chapters on treatment are based on the premise that breast cancer is not a single disease but a spectrum of disease. A reasonably accurate location of the individual patient within this spectrum can be determined after a careful clinical assessment of the patient, combined with a histologic assessment of the tumor. Treatment then varies according to the overall clinical and histologic assessment. A modified mastectomy is the treatment of choice in the majority of cases. In some cases a quadrant excision or subcutaneous mastectomy is feasible, in other cases a radical mastectomy is indicated. Similar principles are outlined in the chapter on the treatment of metastatic breast disease, again emphasizing the need for a treatment regimen based on a comprehensive clinical and histologic assessment.

My thanks to the contributing authors, Doctors Morton L. Levin, David B. Thomas, Joseph C. Eggleston, Darryl Carter, Floyd Osterman, Atsuko Heshiki, and Martin D. Abeloff. I am indepted to Leon Schlossberg for the fine artwork. My secretary, Sharon Sweder, has worked tirelessly on the manuscript and coordinated the entire project. I am most grateful for her invaluable help.

INTRODUCTION

In the late summer of 1853, Catherine Wirt Randall, mother and daughter in a prominent Maryland family, sought medical attention for a lump in her breast of uncertain duration.[1] After consultation with America's most renowned doctors she learned that surgery might not, in her physician's words, "be effective but without it lingering death" would be certain. In the fall, doctors performed an operation in her brother's home, where after the administration of chloric ether they removed the tumor. The procedure took three to four hours, but what nineteenth-century Americans called amputation of the breast did little to improve Mrs. Randall's chance for survival. She died in January 1854. In nineteenth-century America, patients with breast cancer usually only sought medical attention with very large tumors which had been present for prolonged periods of time. Limited amputation of the breast was the accepted form of surgical therapy. Even if unfortunate women such as Catherine Randall survived the operation, the tumor usually recurred within a short period of time. Eighty years later another prominent American woman, Charlotte Perkins Gilman, sought medical attention for her breast cancer. Her tumor was deemed inoperable and no palliative therapy was suggested by her physician. The breast cancer continued to progress and cause increasing pain. She purchased some chloroform and later committed suicide, preferring, as she stated earlier, "chloroform to cancer."[2]

A good deal of progress has been made since the deaths of Mrs. Randall in 1854 and Mrs. Gilman in 1930. Screening procedures combining physical examination with mammography or xeroradiography have detected breast cancers at an earlier stage when conventional treatment is more effective. Clinical trials employing these methods of early detection have demonstrated that the death rate from breast cancer can be reduced by earlier detection. Although mass screening of all women over thirty-five is not economically or logistically feasible at the present time, screening of a high-risk group of patients is feasible, and such a high-risk group of patients has been identified by the epidemiologists. The majority of breast cancers, however, continue to be detected by the patient. The treatment of these patients remains controversial, and a good deal of emotional debate continues, unsupported at times by statistically significant clinical data. Current methods of treatment of the typical patient with breast cancer are relatively ineffective and approximately 50 percent of these women will eventually die of the disease. The relative ineffectiveness of treatment at the present time is primarily due to the inability to detect and treat occult metastatic disease rather than failure to control the primary tumor and its regional lymph node metastasis. Significant reductions in mortality rates from breast cancer are dependent, therefore, upon either prevention of the disease, detection of the primary tumor at a stage which is not associated with a significant incidence of distant metastasis, or the development of better methods of clinical management, including the use of surgical adjuvants which are capable of destroying occult metastases.

In this book we have summarized the current trends in the management of breast cancer. The initial chapter is concerned with the epidemiology of breast cancer, particularly as it applies to early detection and the identification of that group of women who are most apt to develop breast cancer. The second chapter is concerned with a discussion of the pathology of breast cancer, with emphasis on a correlation of histologic findings, with prognosis and treatment. The third chapter deals with radiographic procedures which are capable of detecting early breast cancers. The indications and results obtained by mammography and xeroradiography are discussed. The last two chapters deal with treatment, first of the primary breast cancer and then with the management of metastatic or recurrent breast cancer. Treatment remains controversial and should, in our opinion, vary with the histologic type of tumor and extent of disease. All currently available methods of treatment are presented and discussed. Emphasis is placed on the correlation of the overall clinical assessment of the individual patient, with the selection of various modalities of treatment, whether the treatment be directed toward the primary tumor or toward distant metastases.

Breast cancer continues to kill an estimated 35,000 women a year in the United States. We hope to contribute to a better understanding of the disease, optimal treatment of the individual patient, and a modest reduction in the death rate from this dread disease.

References

1. Elizabeth Randall Clunas to Catherine Randall Gittings November 1853-January 1854, Randall Gittings, Clunas. MSS Maryland Historical Society.
2. *Charlotte Perkins Gilman, the Living of Charlotte Perkins Gilman—An Autobiography* (Arno Press, 1972), pp. 333-34.

CURRENT TRENDS IN THE MANAGEMENT OF BREAST CANCER

1. THE EPIDEMIOLOGY OF BREAST CANCER

Morton L. Levin and David B. Thomas

Introduction

Epidemiology may be defined as the study of the distribution of disease, and of factors—such as time, place, or person—which influence its distribution, in human populations. The chief goal of epidemiologic studies is the discovery of etiology or of clues to etiology. Clinicians have always been interested in the characteristic features of persons having a specific disease. For example, females likely to have cholecystitis have traditionally been described as "fair, fat, and forty." If true, these would be epidemiologic features of cholecystitis. For lung cancer, being male and a cigarette smoker are the most characteristic epidemiologic features. These features may also be considered "risk factors," since they indicate factors which increase or decrease the likelihood that an individual will develop the disease. While all truly etiologic factors are risk factors, the converse is not necessarily true. A risk factor may not be causal, but be associated with another unknown factor which is causal. Deliberately or intuitively the clinician utilizes his knowledge of the epidemiologic features of disease in his consideration of differential diagnosis, in deciding which patients should be examined by detection procedures, and in his understanding of the biology of the disease process.

In the United States, breast cancer death rates are nearly one hundred times higher for women than men [1]. Approximately 7 percent of all women in the United States may be expected to develop breast cancer at some time during their lives. In the 3rd

1

National Cancer Survey (Table 1-1), covering about 10 percent of the U.S. population, there were reported (during the three years 1969-71), in both sexes, 24,670 cases of breast cancer, compared with 24,010 cases of lung cancer, the second most frequent malignant tumor. This preponderance of breast cancer occurred in spite of the fact that the disease is largely restricted to one sex; only 192 breast cancer cases were males. Breast cancer is thus certainly the most common cancer in women, and rare in men. For this reason, this chapter deals primarily with cancer of the female breast. A section specifically devoted to cancer of the male breast is presented at the end of the chapter.

Time Trend

The age-adjusted death rate from breast cancer in the United States has remained remarkably constant for many years at about 25 deaths per 100,000 women per year (1). Given a constant incidence rate, this could be interpreted in at least two ways: (a) that our methods of diagnosis and treatment have little effect on mortality, and the recorded death rate is a reflection of the natural course of the disease and an unchanging incidence, or (b) that our methods of diagnosis and treatment reached their maximum efficacy years ago, so that applied to a constant rate of incidence (age-adjusted) there results a constant rate of death. Another interpretation is suggested by the fact that in recent years there is evidence of some increased incidence of breast cancer. This would suggest some improvement in diagnosis and treatment, which, counterbalanced by increased incidence, again results in a fairly constant death rate (2).

Table 1-1.
Cancer Incidence—Average Annual Cases per 100,000 Population U.S. 1969-71, among White and Negro Women (Age Standardized)[a]

Cancer site	White	Negro	Cancer site	White	Negro
All sites	270.3	256.8	Ovary	14.3	10.7
Breast	75.0	57.7	Rectum and		
Colon, except			recto-sig.	10.6	8.8
rectum	29.4	27.8	Pancreas	7.3	9.8
Fundus uteri	21.0	12.1	Stomach	6.8	9.2
Cervix, inv.	15.0	33.8	Bladder	6.2	4.3
Lung	14.4	14.4			

[a]1970 U.S. population as standard. *Source of data:* reference 66.

Risk Factors

The major factors known or suspected to increase or decrease the risk of developing breast cancer in women are listed in Table 1-2. Some have clinical application, others are of interest chiefly as clues to the etiology or to some biological pattern which may explain the occurrence of breast cancer. The factors listed are discussed below.

Geographic/Ethnic Factors

Perhaps the most striking single epidemiologic characteristic of female breast cancer is its high incidence in the western world (Table 1-2, Fig. 1-1). For example, mortality from and incidence of breast cancer in Japanese women is only about one-fifth that of American women. Such geographic and ethnic differences have been the subject of much speculation and several studies, but remain unexplained. That they may be due largely to environmental rather than genetic factors is suggested by the fact that migrants from low- to high-risk countries develop breast cancer at rates intermediate between those of natives of the countries of origin and adoption. Also,

Table 1-2.
Major Risk Factors for Breast Cancer in Women

Factor	Increased risk	Decreased risk
Geographic/ethnic	North American	Japanese
	West European	Taiwanese
		South African—blacks
		Nigeria—blacks
		Indians
Increasing age	Old	Young
Age at first birth	After age 30	Before age 20
Parity	Nulliparity	Parous before age 20
Age at menarche	Before age 13	After age 16
Age at natural menopause	After age 50	Before age 45
Oopherectomy	—	Before age 45
Nutritional	Obesity	—
Ionizing radiation	Ionizing radiation	
Previous cancer	Breast	Cervix
	Endometrium	
	Colon-rectum	
	Salivary gland	
	Ovary	
Familial	Family history of breast cancer	—
Prior benign breast disease	Fibrocystic breast disease (especially with ductal atypia)	—

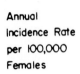

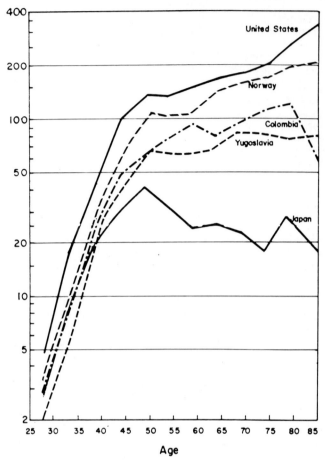

Fig. 1-1. Female breast cancer incidence rate by age, selected areas, periods around 1965.

Note: Colombia (Cali), 1962-66; Japan (averages of Myagi Prefecture, 1962-64, and Okayama Prefecture, 1966); Norway, 1964-66; United States, 1966-68 (estimated, see text); Yugoslavia (Slovenia), 1961-65.

Source of data: reference 4.

rates in succeeding generations tend to approximate those for natives of the country of adoption with the passage of time (1, 3).

Effect of Age

Table 1-3 and Figure 1-1 show that in the United States the incidence of breast cancer rises steeply to age fifty, and then be-

Table 1-3.
Average Annual Breast Cancer Incidence U.S. White Females 1969–1971

Age	Cases per 100,000	Age	Cases per 100,000	Age	Cases per 100,000
20–24	1.1	45–49	159.0	70–74	260.1
25–29	8.7	50–54	171.6	75–79	294.7
30–34	22.4	55–59	191.8	80–84	301.3
35–39	52.5	60–64	226.6	85+	306.8
40–44	103.7	65–69	234.0		

Source of data: reference 66.

comes almost flat for the next five years. After this it increases again, but at a much slower pace (4). The change in the rate of increase at about the age of menopause has been interpreted as indicating that breast cancer occurring after the menopause differs biologically from that occuring up to the menopause and that endogenous hormones are of etiologic importance.

The relationship of breast cancer to age is a complex one. The greatest age effect (in the United States) is between 45 and 49 years, when the incidence increases by about 11 cases per 100,000 for each year of age. Two other high levels of increase occur at ages 60 to 64 and 75 to 79; at both these age-periods there is an increase of almost 7 cases per 100,000 per year of age. At all other ages the increase per year is less than at these three age-periods.

The international differences are greater for women in their postmenopausal than premenopausal years, due to the diminished age effect in the latter type of women in low-risk groups (Fig. 1–1).

Age at First Birth

The age at which a women has her first child is strongly related to her risk of subsequently developing breast cancer (5). The earlier this occurs, the less the risk. Table 1–4, based on data from Boston (6), indicates that women whose first birth occurs before age twenty have less than one-half the breast cancer risk of the general population. Women whose age at first birth is thirty-five years or older have more than 50 percent greater risk than the general population. The risk of breast cancer increases by about 5 percent for each increased year of age at first birth. Nulliparae, with 30 percent greater than general population risk, nevertheless have a lower risk than women with first birth at thirty-five years or over. Risk of breast cancer is only related to early pregnancy that develops to

Table 1-4.
Age at First Birth and Breast Cancer Risk

Age at first birth[a]	% Distribution		Breast cancer risk relative to general population[b]
	Breast cancer	Controls	
< 20	3.1	7.5	.41
20–24	19.6	27.2	.72
25–29	23.4	23.5	1.00
30–34	12.5	10.7	1.17
Nulliparae	35.2	27.0	1.30
35 yrs. +	6.2	4.1	1.51
Total	100.0	100.0	—

a First births include stillbirths at 5 months or older.

b Refers chiefly to women aged 35 and over.

term or to stillbirth at five months or older; it is not related to abortions and miscarriages. These relationships may be interpreted as due to (a) hormonal changes associated with early pregnancy; (b) breast changes so associated, such as preparation for lactation; (c) some other factor or factors which decrease the likelihood of early pregnancy and increase the risk of breast cancer; (d) some combination of these.

Assuming that the relationship between breast cancer risk and age at first birth is causal, and not an indirect statistical one, it can be shown that if all parous women had their first birth before age twenty, and if there were no change in the proportion of nulliparous women (27 percent), then the total breast cancer rate would be decreased by about thirty-five percent. Restriction of childbearing to women under twenty would thus have a smaller effect than oophorectomy at or before age thirty-five, which is discussed subsequently. The latter would decrease breast cancer rates by about 60 percent. Although such procedures are not currently advocated for the general population, these estimates of their effect on the breast cancer problem demonstrate the importance childbearing and ovarian function may have on the genesis of breast cancer. Furthermore, steps such as premenopausal oophorectomy and control of age at first birth may need to be considered in dealing with women who are at high risk of breast cancer, e.g., women with benign breast disease or a family history of breast cancer.

Menstrual Experience

The risk of breast cancer is relatively lower in women with late menarche (7) and early menopause, either artificial (8, 9) or natural (9). (Tables 1-5 and 1-6). Artificial menopause reduces risk only if due to oophorectomy; the amount of risk reduction has been directly related to the amount of resultant ovarian dysfunction and inversely related to the age at which oophorectomy was performed (8). A similar reduction in breast cancer risk has been noted in spayed female dogs, and the amount of reduction is inversely related to the age of the dog at surgery (10).

Lactation Experience

Because lactation effectively inhibits ovarian function, it is reasonable to wonder whether breast feeding, like oophorectomy, reduces the risk of breast cancer. The results of studies that deal with this question are inconsistent, but the largest and more comprehensive one showed no relationship between lactation and breast cancer (11). If lactation has a protective effect, it is weak, limited to women who lactate for periods that are prolonged by U.S. standards, and not the explanation for geographic and ethnic differences in breast cancer rates. The significant factor may be the age at which the breast is first developed to lactation capability.

Endogenous Hormones

The fact that women have much higher rates of breast cancer than men, the observation that the rate of change of incidence with age is

Table 1-5.
Relative Risk of Breast Cancer in Women with Natural Menopause at Various Ages

Age at menopause	Relative risk [a]
< 45	0.73
45–49	0.93
50–54	1.07
55+	1.48

[a] Risk relative to that of women having natural menopause between age 45 and 54 years.
Source of data: reference 9.

Table 1–6.
Relative Risk of Breast Cancer in Women with Oophorectomy at Various Ages

Age of oophorectomy	Relative risk[a]
< 35	0.36
35–39	0.68
40–44	0.65
45–49	0.73
50 and older	0.98

a Risk relative to that of women with natural menopause at age 45–54 years.
Source of data: reference 9.

different for pre- and postmenopausal women, and the associations between breast cancer and woman's childbearing and menstrual experiences, all suggest that endogenous sex hormones may play a role in the genesis of breast cancer. This hypothesis is strengthened by the observation that males with breast cancer tend to have a prior history of orchitis, orchiectomy, and treatment with hormones (12).

The nature of the hormonal aberrations that lead to breast cancer is not well understood. A number of studies have been conducted in which levels of various hormones in blood or urine from cases and controls were compared. Such studies have largely led to inconsistent results that are difficult to interpret. A major problem with them is that the presence of the breast tumor may itself cause abnormal hormonal patterns. To avoid this, studies have been conducted in which either hormonal patterns in tumor-free individuals at relatively high and low risk of breast cancer were compared, or hormonal patterns in normal women were ascertained and then the women were followed over time to determine the relationship of the observed patterns to the subsequent development of breast cancer. To date, all such hormonal studies have been based on measurements of urinary metabolities of estrogens or androgens. This limits interpretation of results because the relationship between patterns of excretion of such metabolities and levels of them or their precursors in blood and breast tissue are unclear, and because the interrelationships between various hormones are not well understood. Nonetheless, some of these studies have provided the basis for both current etiologic theories and subsequent ongoing investigations. For these reasons, selected results of some investigations are briefly summarized below.

It has been shown that compared to British women the Japanese, who represent a relatively low-risk population, excrete more of their (adrenal produced) androgens as the active compound androsterone and less as the inactive aetiocholanolone. Also, a prospective study of initially normal women on the Isle of Guernsey has shown the incidence of breast cancer to be inversely related to the urinary levels of either of these substances as measured from five months to nine years prior to the development of clinical disease (13). In addition, sisters of the women who developed breast cancer on Guernsey, as well as women with benign breast disease (two groups at high risk of breast cancer), also excreted subnormal levels of these androgen metabolites (14). Thus, urinary excretion of low levels of androgen metabolities and excretion of the inactive form of such substances are associated with an increased risk of breast cancer.

The three major estrogen fractions excreted in urine are estrone, estradiol, and estriol. The first two are estrogenically active and carcinogenic in mice; the third is estrogenically inactive and can inhibit the carcinogenic effect of estrone in mice (15). Lemon (16) has hypothesized that a high ratio of urinary estriol to estrone plus estradiol (the urinary estriol excretion ratio) should be associated with a decreased risk of breast cancer in women. This is consistent with the knowledge that a low estriol excretion ratio is associated with such risk factors for breast cancer as early menarche, low fertility, and delayed first pregnancy (17). Furthermore, the protective factor, premenopausal oophorectomy, is associated with a high estriol excretion rates (17). More importantly, low-risk Asian women have been shown to have higher ratios than relatively higher-risk North American women; and women of Japanese and Chinese descent in Hawaii, who have intermediate rates of breast cancer, have intermediate ratios (18, 19). The urinary estriol excretion ratio is thus inversely associated with breast cancer risk in humans.

These associations between patterns of urinary excretion of androgen and estrogen metabolities may not in themselves be etiologic. However, they are indicators of endocrinologic abnormalities at the breast tissue level, which may play a role in the genesis of breast cancer. The etiology of such abnormalities is unknown, but they could be ovarian, pituitary, adrenal, or mammary in origin. Much more work to elucidate interrelationships between various hormones and associations between urinary metabolities and tissue levels of these or their precursors needs to be done before the relation of endogenous hormones to the risk of breast cancer can be understood.

Nutrition

Geographic differences in the incidence of breast cancer, and the fact that migrants from low- to high-risk countries develop breast cancer at rates similar or close to rates in the country of adoption with the passage of time, suggest that environmental factors play a role in the genesis of breast cancer. At least some of these factors may be dietary. Rates of breast cancer in various countries are positively correlated with mean annual per capita consumption of sugar, protein, and fat (20). Both a high-fat diet and obesity have been particularly implicated. A high-fat diet increased the proportion of DMBA treated rats that developed breast tumors (21), and, compatible with the endogenous hormone hypothesis, it has been noted that a high-fat diet increases the amount of biliary steroids (cholesterol and bile-salt degradation products) in feces and also renders the intraintestinal environment more favorable to the growth of anaerobic lecithinase-negative clostridia (22). In vitro, these organisms can produce estrone, estradiol, and 17-methoxy-oestradiol from cholestenone, a bacterial metabolite of cholesterol that is present in feces.

Breast cancer has been directly related to obesity (23), particularly in postmenopausal women (24). After menopause, estrogens are produced by the conversion of androstenedione, which is of adrenal cortical origin, to estrone; this conversion takes place primarily in adipose tissue, and more readily in obese women (25). Thus, like the various reproductive factors previously discussed, obesity and dietary fat could also be related to breast cancer development because of associated changes in endogenous hormones.

Exogenous Hormones

The evidence that endogenous hormones are somehow related to the development of breast cancer has naturally suggested that exogenous hormones might be carcinogenic. Of the various classes of exogenous estrogen preparations, the oral contraceptives are of particular concern, because their use is widespread and they are taken primarily by women in their early menstrual years, when the relative levels of endogenous estrogens are hypothesized to alter the risk of breast cancer (5). Estrogens used for replacement therapy at menopause are also of great concern. Because early cessation of ovarian function is protective, it is reasonable to wonder whether effectively prolonging the premenopausal period by artificial means might enhance breast tumor development.

However, although high doses of estrogens have resulted in the development of mammary tumors in experimental animals (26) and male transsexuals (27), little evidence is available to date that implicates steroidal oral contraceptives or preparations used for menopause as mammary carcinogens.

Seven studies of this question have now reported no increased risk of breast cancer among women taking oral contraceptives. Several studies report also a decreased association of fibrocystic disease in this group (74-80).

The absence of a proven relationship between exogenous estrogens and breast cancer should nonetheless be interpreted with some caution. Most known carcinogenic agents produce tumors only after a long latency period, and insufficient time may have elapsed since exogenous sources of estrogens were first used for manifestation of their carcinogenic effect. For this reason a number of studies are being continued to further investigate the relationship between steroidal preparations and breast cancer.

Viral Hypothesis

Recent biochemical and virologic studies have provided strong evidence that an oncogenic RNA virus with properties similar to those of the mouse mammary tumor virus may be involved in the genesis of breast cancer in women (28, 29). Epidemiologic studies, however, have clearly shown that having been breast fed as an infant, either by a mother who subsequently developed breast cancer or by one who did not, does not alter ones risk of mammary carcinoma (30-33). This does not invalidate the laboratory evidence for a viral etiology, but it does indicate that any human mammary tumor virus that may ultimately be identified is not transmitted in an oncogenic form via breast milk.

The epidemiologic features of breast cancer previously described must also be explained when considering a viral etiology. There are two possible interpretations. One is that the virus may by itself cause breast cancer, but only a small proportion of all cases. This seems unlikely because several laboratory studies based on small numbers of cases have consistently shown evidence for a mammary tumor virus. The other interpretation is that the virus is widespread, but does not by itself cause cancer; rather it is only oncogenic under the proper (hormonal?) conditions. Much additional work needs to be done before the results of all laboratory and epidemiologic studies render a clear understanding of the role viruses may play in the etiology of breast cancer.

Ionizing Radiation

There is strong evidence that high doses of ionizing radiation can cause breast cancer. Survivors of the atomic bomb explosions in Japan who received 90 rads or more of radiation subsequently developed breast cancer at a rate two to four times that for nonexposed individuals (34). Women who received multiple fluoroscopic examinations in the course of artificial pneumothorax treatment for pulmonary tuberculosis had an incidence of breast cancer that was nine times greater than that for tuberculosis patients not so treated (35). In the former group the breast cancer occurred on the same side of the body as the pneumothorax, and there was a clear relationship between dose of radiation as measured by number of fluoroscopies and incidence of disease.

However, few women are subjected to the amount of radiation comparable to that received by women in these studies, and such exposure can therefore account for only a small proportion of all breast cancer cases. The effect of such low doses of radiation as received from chest X-rays and mammography on breast cancer development has not been studied directly, but must be considered in evaluating the risks of mammography.

Other Malignancies

Women who have had breast cancer are at greatly increased risk of developing a second neoplasm of the opposite breast (36, 37). There is some increased risk also of cancer of the colon, rectum, pancreas, bronchus, lung, ovary, and endometrium (36, 38, 39); and women with carcinomas of the salivary gland, colon, rectum, ovary, and endometrium are more prone than normal women to develop breast cancer (Table 1-2) (36, 40-44). It is unknown whether these associations are due to etiologic factors in the environment that are common to various neoplasms, due to a nonspecific increased susceptibility to cancer in some individuals, or due to a direct influence of one cancer on the development of another.

Women with carcinoma of the uterine cervix are at low risk of breast cancer, and vice versa. The explanation for this negative association probably lies in the fact that risk of the former neoplasm is inversely related to age at first sexual intercourse, while risk of the latter is directly related to age at first pregnancy.

Hereditary or Familial Factors

Most family studies of breast cancer show that there is roughly a twofold frequency of breast cancer among mothers and sisters of breast cancer patients (45). Also, studies of families in which two or more women developed breast cancer have shown that other members of such families are at increased risk of developing cancer of the colon, stomach, ovary, endometrium, and brain, as well as sarcomas and leukemia (46).

While these associations could be due to either hereditary or common environmental factors, there is additional evidence that heredity may play a role in the genesis of at least some mammary carcinomas: relatives of women with bilateral disease and disease of early onset appear to be at particularly high risk (47); it has been reported that the rate of breast cancer in blacks has been correlated with the frequency of the Duffy allele "Fy^a," which is a measure of the amount of Caucasian genetic mixture in the population (48); breast cancer has been reported to be associated with blood type as in the MNS-antigen system (49), types A and O in the ABO system (50) and HL-A7 of the major histocompatibility system; men with Klinefelter's syndrome have a high incidence of gynecomastia and perhaps an increased risk of breast cancer (51); and there is some evidence for an aberrant no. 2 chromosome in breast cancer patients with a family history of breast cancer, and in their relatives (52).

However, great caution must be exercised in interpreting these findings. Not all family studies show familial aggregation; the chromosomal aberration was observed in only a small number of study subjects with incompletely verified family histories; and the associations between breast cancer and blood types as in the MNS-system, and A and O in the ABO system, as well as the associations with Duffy blood group and HL-47 antigen, have not been consistently demonstrated by all investigators and tend to be weak when observed.

There is definitely a need for further family studies of breast cancer to more clearly elucidate the role hereditary factors may play in its genesis.

Benign Breast Disease

Belief in a relation of fibrocystic breast disease to increased risk of breast cancer is widely held, although not definitely established (53). For example, the text *Clinical Oncology* (edited by the Committee on Professional Education of UICC [Springer-Verlag; Berlin–Heidelberg 1973]) states: "The presence of cystic disease of the breast seems to be a factor predisposing to breast cancer, the incidence of the latter among patients with the former being two to three times that of the general population." A recent review (68) of a study of 1,000 breast cancer cases, found proliferative fibrocystic disease (intraductal papillomatosis and lobular hyperplasia) in the "vicinity or quadrant" of the malignant mass in 34.9 percent of cases, and the nonproliferative form (fibrosis, cysts, sclerosing adenosis, blunt duct adenosis, and apocrine change) in 20.6 percent.

The most recent study, from the Mayo Clinic (69), provides evidence that among women who had previously had either local resection or mastectomy for fibrocystic disease there occurred, during a 13.5 year follow-up period, almost three times the number of breast cancer cases which would be expected, based on the incidence of breast cancer in the general female population of Rochester, Minnesota. The relation of fibrocystic disease to subsequent breast cancer incidence remains equivocal, in part because of differences in the pathologic characterization of fibrocystic disease, but cannot be excluded as a distinct possibility. The presence of atypical ductal cells indicates a particularly high risk of carcinoma (54, 67). Lobular carcinoma in siter and intraductal papillomatosis are considered to be precancerous lesions.

Reserpine

Treatment of hypertension with the rauwolfia alkaloid, reserpine, has been reported to increase the risk of breast cancer. Three case-control studies have reported a 2.0- to 3.5-fold increased risk of breast cancer among users of reserpine (55–57). Since these three studies employed somewhat different designs and were conducted in different countries by different investigators, the consistency of the results suggests that they are not spurious, although the methods used in each individual study have been criticized. Hypertension treated by other medication was not associated with breast cancer.

Reserpine could theoretically alter the risk of breast cancer in at least three ways: (a) by stimulation of prolactin, which in rodents enhances the growth of mammary tumors induced by DMBA (58);

(b) by immunologic suppression, since reserpine suppresses delayed hypersensitivity, which may influence breast tumor growth and metastasis (59, 60); and (c) by serving as a precursor of a chemical carcinogen. Reserpine is excreted in human milk (61), and metabolities of reserpine are chemically similar to some compounds known to induce nasal squamous cell carcinoma in rats, as well as to others that may have caused mammary and hepatic tumors in mice (62).

Although it cannot be stated with certainty that reserpine can cause breast cancer in women, the possibility exists. Additional epidemiologic studies to answer these questions have now been reported. In three of these (70, 71, 72), no relationship between the use of reserpine or rauwolfia derivatives has been found. In the fourth study (73), again no clear evidence of a relationship was found. The authors note, however, that "a small effect may not have been detected in the studies reporting negative results." They suggest that "it is also possible that a sub-group of women with characteristics that have been previously found to be associated with breast cancer, such as early age at first birth, early menarche, late menopause, and certain hormonal profiles, may be at a higher risk of developing breast cancer if given reserpine" (73).

Breast Cancer in Males

Like female rates, the mortality rates of breast cancer in males increase with age. Furthermore, the change in the rate of increase with age, although not as great as in females, is also noted in males (12). This suggests that factors other than endocrine changes at menopause may influence the age trend in women.

Married men have lower rates of breast cancer than single, divorced or widowed men, as is true for women. However, among the unmarried, the rates for widowed or divorced men are higher than for single men, whereas the opposite is true for women (12). One theoretical mechanism that could account for the marital difference in males is that divorced and widowed males are known to have a higher frequency of alcoholic liver cirrhosis than married men. Pathological changes in the liver impair the excretion of endogenous estrogens, resulting in gynecomastia, which has been related to male breast cancer.

The same international differences in rates of female breast cancer have also been noted for males. Rates for both sexes are low in Japan, for example. This suggests that the environmental factors responsible for the difference in rates of predominantly postmenopausal breast cancer in females may also be of importance in males.

Although of a different nature than for females, studies have implicated hormones also in the genesis of male breast cancer. Compared to controls, male breast cancer patients have a more frequent prior history of orchitis, orchiectomy, treatment with hormones (thyroid, cortisone, testosterone, or stilbestrol), and gynecomastia (63). Male transsexuals treated with high doses of estrogens to stimulate mammary growth have developed breast cancer (27). Men with Klinefelter's syndrome have both testicular disorders and gynecomastia, and estimates indicate that such men have a risk of breast cancer that is about one-fifth that of women, representing about twenty times the normal male rate (64). It has been suggested that the relatively high incidence of breast cancer among males in Egypt reflects the high prevalence of liver damage due to bilharziasis (65). The relationship of male breast cancer to alcoholic cirrhosis in western countries has not been studied.

Like the female relatives of women with breast cancer, male relatives of afflicted men also more frequently develop breast cancer than do relatives of unaffected controls (12). This indicates that the factor responsible for familial aggregation of breast cancer is not a sex-linked inherited trait.

Ionizing radiation increases the risk of male as well as of female breast cancer (12).

Summary and Conclusions

Present knowledge of the epidemiology of breast cancer does not as yet provide an adequate pattern to fully explain why some women do and others do not develop the disease. Nevertheless, the epidemiologic observations do suggest the possibility of application in two areas: primary prevention (prevention of occurrence) and secondary prevention (prevention of fatal outcome by screening and early diagnosis followed by definitive treatment).

For primary prevention of breast cancer, the possibility of control is suggested by (a) the relation to age at first birth, if indeed this relation proves to be causal rather than selective, and (b) the relationship to oophorectomy before age thirty-five. For the latter relationship, the evidence for a truly preventive effect is fairly clear. Avoiding reserpine treatment for hypertension and controlling obesity in postmenopausal women also present possible areas of prevention, if further study confirms these apparent relationships.

For secondary prevention (screening), the importance of considering high-risk factors is emphasized by the practical impossibility of screening all women aged thirty-five years and over as often as once a year. The screening centers now in operation cannot always screen all those who apply, and the numbers of those applying probably will continue to increase. A hierarchy of preferred characteristics for screening would include women (a) of increasing age, (b) with a familial history of breast cancer, (c) with fibrocystic breast disease, (d) whose first live birth occurred after age thirty, (e) who are nulliparae, (f) whose menarche occurred before age thirteen years, and (g) whose menopause occurred after age fifty. As the enthusiasm for breast cancer screening increases, some selection of preferred subjects for screening will be needed.

References

1. Lilienfeld, A. M., Levin, M. L., and Kessler, I. I. 1972. *Cancer in the United States.* Harvard University Press.
2. Cutler, S. J., Christine, B., and Barclay, T. H. C. 1971. Increasing incidence and decreasing mortality rates for breast cancer. *Cancer* 25:1376–80.
3. Buell, P. 1973. Changing incidence of breast cancer in Japanese-American women. *J. Natl. Cancer Inst.* 51:1479–83.
4. Seidman, H. 1973. *Cancer of the breast. Statistical and epidemiological data.* Am. Cancer Soc. Professional Education Publication.
5. MacMahon, B., Cole, P., Brown, J. B. 1973. Etiology of human breast cancer. *J. Natl. Cancer Inst.* 50:21–42.
6. MacMahon, B., Cole, P., Lin, T. M., et al. 1970. Age at first birth and breast cancer. *Bull. Wld. Hlth. Org.* 43:209–21.
7. Staszewski, J. 1971. Age at menarche and breast cancer. *J. Natl. Cancer Inst.* 47:935–40.
8. Hirayama, T., Wynder, E. L. 1962. A study of the epidemiology of cancer of the breast. II. The influence of hysterectomy. *Cancer* 15:28–38.
9. Trichopoulos, D., MacMahon, B., Cole, P. 1972. Menopause and breast cancer risk. *J. Natl. Cancer Inst.* 48:605–13.
10. Schneider, R., Dorn, C. R., Taylor, D. O. N. 1969. Factors influencing canine mammary cancer development and postsurgical survival. *J. Natl. Cancer Inst.* 43:1249–61.
11. MacMahon, B., Lin, T. M., Lowe, C. R., et al. 1969. Lactation and cancer of the breast. A summary of an international study. *Bull. Wld. Hlth. Org.* 42:1249–61.
12. Scottenfeld, D., and Lilienfeld, A. M. 1963. Some epidemiological features of breast cancer among males. *J. Chron. Dis.* 16:71–81.
13. Bulbrook, R. D., Hayward, J. L., and Spicer, C. C. 1971. Relation between urinary androgen and corticoid execretion and subsequent breast cancer. *Lancet* 2:395–98.
14. Brennan, M. J., Bulbrook, R. D., Deshpande, H., et al. 1973. Urinary and plasma androgens in benign breast disease. *Lancet* 1:1076–79.
15. Pullinger, B. 1961. Increase in mammary carcinoma and adenocarcinoma and incidence of other tumors in C3HF virgin females after ovariectomy and high doses with some oestrogens. *Brit. J. Cancer* 15:574–83.
16. Lemon, H. M. 1970. Abnormal estrogen metabolism and tissue estrogen receptor proteins in breast cancer. *Cancer* 25:423–35.
17. Sherman, B. M., and Korenman, S. G. 1974. Inadequate corpus luteum function: A pathophysiological interpretation of human breast cancer epidemiology. *Cancer* 33:1306–12.

18. Dickinson, L. E., MacMahon, B., Cole, P., et al. 1974. Estrogen profiles of oriental and caucasian women in Hawaii. New Engl. J. Med. 291:1211-13.

19. MacMahon, B., Cole, P., Brown, J. B., et al. 1974. Urine oestrogen profiles of Asian and North American women. Int. J. Cancer 14:161-67.

20. Draser, B. S., Irving, D. 1973. Environmental factors and cancer of the colon and breast. Brit. J. Cancer 27:167-72.

21. Carroll, K. K., Gammal, E. B., Plunkett, E. R. 1968. Dietary fat and mammary cancer. Can. Med. Assoc. J. 98:590-94.

22. Hill, M. J., Goddard, P., Williams, R. E. O. 1971. Gut bacteria and aetiology of cancer of the breast. Lancet 2:472-73.

23. Wynder, E. L., Bross, I. J., and Hirayama, T. 1960. A study of the epidemiology of cancer of the breast. Cancer 13:559-601.

24. DeWaard, F., Baanders-van Halewijn, E. A., and Huizinga, J. 1964. The bimodal age distribution of patients with mammary carcinoma. Evidence for the existence of 2 types of human breast cancer. Cancer 17:141-51.

25. Kirschner, M. 1974. Relation of endocrine functions to epidemiological characteristics of breast cancer. Presented at Breast Cancer Task Force "Report to the Profession" Meeting. September 30, 1974. National Institutes of Health, Bethesda, Maryland, U.S.A.

26. Shubik, P., and Hartwell, J. L. 1957. Survey of compounds which have been tested for carcinogenic activity. Publication 149, suppl. 1, U.S. Public Health Service, pp. 250-57.

27. Symmers, W. S. 1968. Carcinoma of the breast in transsexual individuals after surgical and hormonal interference with the primary and secondary sex characteristics. Brit. Med. J.. 2:83-85.

28. Schlom, J., and Spiegelman, S. 1974. Breast cancer. Molecular basis for a viral etiology. N.Y. State J. Med. 74:1373-84.

29. Moore, D. H. 1974. Evidence in favor of the existence of human breast cancer virus. Cancer Res. 34:2322-29.

30. Bucalossi, P., and Veronesi, U. 1959. Researches on the etiological factors in human breast cancer. Acta Union Internationale Contre Le Cancer 15:1056-60.

31. Henderson, B. E. 1974. Type B virus and human breast cancer. Cancer 34:1386-89.

32. Morgan, R. W., Vakil, D. V., and Chipman, M. L. 1974. Breast feeding, family history, and breast disease. Amer. J. Epidemiol. 99:117-22.

33. Tokuhata, G. K. 1969. Morbidity and mortality among offspring of breast cancer mothers. Amer. J. Epidemiol. 89:139-53.

34. Wanebo, C. K., Johnson, K. G., Sato, K., et al. 1968. Breast cancer after exposure to the atomic bombings of Hiroshima and Nagasaki. New Engl. J. Med. 279:667-71.

35. Myrden, J. A., Hiltz, J. E. 1969. Breast cancer following multiple fluoroscopies during artificial pneumothorax treatment of pulmonary tuberculosis. Can. Med. Assoc. J. 100:1032-34.

36. Schottenfeld, D., Berg, J. 1971. Incidence of multiple primary cancers. IV. Cancers of the female breast and genital organs. J. Natl. Cancer Inst. 46:161-70.

37. Lewison, E. F., Neto, A. S. 1971. Bilateral breast cancer at the Johns Hopkins Hospital. Cancer 28:1297-1201.

38. Schoenberg, B. S., Greenberg, R. A., Eisenberg, H. 1969. Occurrence of certain multiple primary cancers in females. J. Natl. Cancer Inst. 43:15-32.

39. Robertson, J., Matthews, V. L., Barclay, T. H. C. 1973. Subsequent primary malignancies in Saskatchewan women with breast cancer. Presented at 1973 Annual Meeting of Society for Epidemiological Research.

40. Schottenfeld, D., Berg, J., Vitsky, B. 1969. Incidence of multiple primary cancers II. Index carriers arising in the stomach and lower digestive system. J. Natl. Cancer Inst. 43:77-86.

41. Berg, J. W., Hutter, R. V. P., Foote, F. W. 1968. The unique association between salivary gland cancer and breast cancer. JAMA 204:771-74.

18   MORTON L. LEVIN AND DAVID B. THOMAS

42. Dunn, J. E., Bragg, K. U., Sautter, C., et al. 1972. Breast cancer risk following a major salivary gland carcinoma. *Cancer* 29:1343-46.
43. Vongtama, V., Kurohara, S. S., Badib, A. O., et al. 1970. Second primary cancers of endometrial carcinoma. *Cancer* 26:842-46.
44. MacMahon, B., Austin, J. H. 1969. Association of carcinomas of the breast and corpus uteri. *Cancer* 23:275-80.
45. Lilienfeld, A. M. 1963. The epidemiology of breast cancer. *Cancer Res.* 23:1503-13.
46. Lynch, H. T., Krush, A. J., Lemon, H. M., et al 1972. Tumor variation in families with breast cancer. *JAMA* 222:1631-35.
47. Anderson, D. E. 1971. Some characteristics of familial breast cancer. *J. Am. Cancer Soc.* 28:1500-04.
48. Zippin, C., Petrakis, N. L. 1971. Identification of high risk groups in breast cancer. *J. Am. Cancer Soc.* 28:1381-87.
49. Report from Boston Collaborative Drug Surveillance Program. 1971. Relation between breast cancer and S blood-antigen system. *Lancert* 1:301-04.
50. Vogel, F. 1970. BO blood groups and disease. *Am. J. Human Genet.* 22:464-75.
51. Harnden, D. G., MacLean, N., Langlands, A. O. 1971. Carcinoma of the breast and Klinefelter's syndrome. *J. Med. Genetics* 8:460-61.
52. Merz, T., El-Mahdi, A. M., Prempree, T. 1968. Unusual chromosomes and malignant disease. *Lancet* 1:337-39.
53. Warren, S. 1940. The relation of "chronic mastitis" to carcinoma of the breast. *Surg. Gynecol. Obstet.* 71:257-73.
54. Black, M. M., Barclay, T. H., Cutler, S. J., et al. 1972. Association of atypical characteristics of benign breast lesions with subsequent risk of breast cancer. *Cancer* 29: 338-43.
55. Boston Collaborative Drug Surveillance Program. 1974. Reserpine and breast cancer. *Lancet* 2:669-71.
56. Armstrong, B., Stevens, N., and Doll, R. 1974. Retrospective study of the association between use of rauwolfia derivatives and breast cancer in women. *Lancet* 2:672-75.
57. Heinonen, O. P., Shipiro, S., Tuominen, L., et al. 1975. Reserpine use in relation to breast cancer. *Lancet* 2:675-77.
58. Welsch, C. W., and Meites, J. 1970. Effects of reserpine on development of 7,12-dimethylbenzanthracene induced mammary tumors. *Experientia* 26:1133-34.
59. Black, M. M. 1973. Human breast cancer. A model for cancer immunology. *Israel J. Med. Sci.* 9:284.
60. Cazenave, J., Reimers, H., Perey, D. Y. E., et al. 1974. Rauwolfia derivatives and breast cancer. *Lancet* 2:1571-72.
61. O'Brien, T. E. 1974. Excretion of drugs in human milk. *Am. J. Hosp. Pharm.* 31:844-54.
62. Schoental, R. 1974. Are rauwolfia alkaloids carcinogenic? *Lancet* 2:1571.
63. Schottenfeld, D., and Lilienfeld, A. M. 1963. Some observations on the epidemiology of breast cancer among males. *Amer. J. Publ. Hlth.* 53:890-96.
64. Scheike, O., Visfeldt, J., and Petersen, B. 1973. Male breast cancer. 3. Breast carcinoma in association with the Klinefelter's syndrome. *Acta Path. Microbiol. Scand.*, section A. 81:352-58.
65. El-Gazayerli, M. M., and Abdel-Aziz, A. S. 1964. On bilharziasis and male breast cancer in Egypt: A preliminary report and review of the literature. *Brit. J. Cancer* 17:566-71.
66. *The Third National Cancer Survey: Advanced Three Year Report, 1969-1971 Incidence*—DHEW Pub. No. (NIH) 74-637 February 1, 1974.
67. Leis, H. P., Jr. 1970. *Diagnosis and treatment of breast lesions.* Flushing, N.Y.: Medical Examination Pub. Co., pp. 79-82.
68. Fisher, E. R., et al. 1975. The pathology of invasive breast cancer. *Cancer* 36:1-85.

69. Donnelly, P. K., Baker, K. W., Carney, J. A., and O'Fallon, W. M. 1975. Benign breast lesions and subsequent breast carcinoma in Rochester, Minnesota. *Mayo Clin. Pro.* 50:650-56.
70. Mack, T. M., Henderson, B. E., Gerkins, V. R., Arthur, M., Bapista, J., and Pike, M. C. 1975. Reserpine and breast cancer in a retirement community. *N. Engl. J. Med.* 292:1366.
71. O'Fallon, W. M., Labarthe, D. R., and Kurland, L. T. 1975. Rauwolfia derivatives and breast cancer: A case control study in Olmstead County, Minnesota. *Lancet* 2:292.
72. Laska, E. M., Siegel, C., Meisner, M., Fischer, S., and Wanderling, J. 1975. Matched-pairs study of reserpine use and breast cancer. *Lancet* 2:296.
73. Lilienfeld, A. M., Chang, L., and Thomas, D. B. 1976. Rauwolfia derivatives and breast cancer. Submitted for publication, April 18, 1976.
74. Vessey, M. P., Doll, R., Sutton, P. M. 1972. Oral contraceptives and breast neoplasia: A retrospective study. *Brit. Med. J.* 3:719-24.
75. Sartwell, P. E., Arthes, F. G., Tonascia, J. A. 1973. Epidemiology of benign breast lesions: Lack of association with oral contraceptive use. *New Engl. J. Med.* 288:551-54.
76. Boston Collaborative Drug Surveillance Program. 1973. Oral contraceptives and venous thromboembolic disease, surgically confirmed gall bladder disease, and breast tumors. *Lancet* 1:1399-1404.
77. Kelsey, J. L., Lindfors, K. K., White, C. 1974. A case-control study of the epidemiology of benign breast diseases with reference to oral contraceptive use. *Int. J. Epidemiol.* 3:333-40.
78. Vessey, M. P., Doll, R., Jones, K. 1975. Oral contraceptives and breast cancer: Progress report of an epidemiological study. *Lancet* 1:941-44.
79. Fasal, E., Paffenbarger, R. S., Jr. 1975. Oral contraceptives as related to cancer and benign lesions of the breast. *J. Natl. Cancer Inst.* 55:767-73.
80. Ory, H., Cole, P., MacMahon, B., Hoover, R. 1976. Oral contraceptives and reduced risk of benign breast diseases. *New Engl. J. Med.* 294:419-22.

2. THE PATHOLOGY OF BREAST CANCER

Darryl Carter and Joseph C. Eggleston

The majority of breast cancers are detected by the patient who feels a mass in her breast. The detection of the mass leads to an examination by a physician, usually followed by hospitalization and a varying number of laboratory procedures and X-rays designed to assess the patient's general condition and to detect distant metastases. Following this evaluation, the patient undergoes either an excisional or incisional biopsy and a specimen is delivered to the surgical pathologist. Any further therapeutic maneuvers are delayed until the pathologist has made a histologic diagnosis. A histologic diagnosis is established either by a frozen section or from material embedded in paraffin. A frozen section diagnosis can be rendered in about fifteen minutes; preparation of sections from paraffin blocks usually takes about twenty-four hours.

The clinical management of a patient with a breast mass is described in detail in Chapter 4. The clinical indications for a breast biopsy fall into two general categories: (1) the patient has a palpable mass in the breast, or (2) a nonpalpable lesion is detected by either mammogram or xerogram.

The majority of discrete breast masses can be biopsied under local anesthesia, thus eliminating the need for a frozen section diagnosis, other than to reassure the patient as to the nature of the lesion. The reasons for this approach are discussed in Chapter 4.

If the patient has the clinical signs of a malignant tumor and is not concerned with the possibility of waking up without her breast, a breast biopsy under general anesthesia, frozen section and imme-diate mastectomy is a reasonable approach to clinical management.

Frozen Sections

If the surgeon and the patient decide to proceed with this ap-proach, the biopsy is obtained directly from the operating room by a member of the pathology staff, who discusses the specific details of the case with the surgeon. The biopsy specimen is brought into the pathology laboratory where it is examined by a pathologist. The gross examination of the tissue is of critical importance. It is thoroughly sectioned at 2 to 3 mm intervals in order to expose a maximum surface area. Since the pathologist is searching for an invasive carcinoma, most of which have a scirrhous reaction, pal-pation of the entire biopsy is of great importance.

The portion of the biopsy which is most suggestive of cancer is selected by the pathologist for frozen section. This is frozen in liquid nitrogen for about 45 seconds so that a thin $(6\text{-}10\mu)$ section may be cut from it in a cryostat. (A cryostat is essentially a sharp knife with a microtome of the type used to cut sections for paraffin blocks. The entire apparatus is enclosed in a refrigerated box at -20°C.) The section is placed on a glass slide, stained with hematoxylin and eosin, and mounted for microscopic examination.

A good histologic preparation is obtained with this technique and the pathologist is able to accurately classify almost all breast lesions on frozen section. The limitations of the frozen section technique are those of sampling error and thickness. It is not practical to freeze and cut more than a few blocks of tissue while the patient is under general anesthesia so that grossly inapparent lesions (such as in situ carcinomas) may not be detected at the time of frozen section. Also, in lesions where cellularity is critical to the diagnosis (such as lobular carcinoma in situ or the unusual papillary lesion), the vari-ability and thickness of the slide may be a hindrance. These limita-tions are not a hindrance to the rapid histological identification of invasive carcinomas, but they do hinder the pathologist in the iden-tification of preinvasive cancer. After the frozen section diagnosis has been made, eight blocks of tissue from each biopsy are submitted for processing into paraffin and sections from these become avail-able the next day. They are examined for the presence of in situ car-cinoma. Microscopic examination of the permanent histologic sec-tions is one of the most effective methods of early detection, since it is relatively inexpensive, and it is the only reliable method of detecting a preinvasive lesion. As previously noted, the limitations of the frozen section technique are not related to histologic identification of an invasive cancer but are related to sampling error and thickness. These limitations of sampling error and thickness of the section are another reason to perform a breast biopsy under local anesthesia, particularly if there is some doubt as to the clinical diagnosis. This approach allows the pathologist to examine permanent histologic sections of all of the tissue prior to any clinical decision as to further management.

If the sole indication for a breast biopsy is an abnormality detected by a mammogram or xeroradiogram, the clinical approach is modified. Breast biopsies performed for these clinically occult but X-ray-suspicious lesions are usually performed under general anesthesia, because the operation can last for prolonged periods of time and larger amounts of tissue must be removed in order to insure removal of the radiographic abnormality. The operation is solely designed to excise the lesion; a histologic diagnosis can be made after examination of permanent histologic sections.

A suspicious lesion detected by a xeroradiogram is carefully localized with the radiologist prior to operation (see Chapter 3). It is then excised and a xeroradiogram of the biopsy specimen is obtained, confirming the presence of the lesion. The incision is closed and the specimen sent to the pathology laboratory, where permanent histologic sections are prepared. A frozen section diagnosis is not always reliable, since these lesions are usually not palpable and the pathologist cannot always determine which area to examine with the frozen section technique.

Lesions detected by a preoperative mammogram are excised in a similar fashion. The biopsy specimen is then examined by a small X-ray unit in the pathology laboratory to confirm the presence of the X-ray abnormality. Permanent histologic sections are then obtained. In our experience, the presence or absence of the X-ray abnormality is much more accurately confirmed by a xeroradiogram of the specimen than it is by a mammogram of the specimen.

The majority of patients who undergo breast biopsy do not have carcinoma; they have some type of cystic disease with proliferative activity. In our experience, the ratio of biopsies for a mass in the breast due to cystic disease with varying degrees of proliferative activity to those which are carcinoma is approximately four to one. The ratio is higher in premenopausal women than in postmenopausal women.

Cystic Disease with Proliferative Activity

Cystic disease with proliferative activity is associated with a broad spectrum of changes. These histologic changes can be consi dered as four types which are certainly not mutually exclusive. These types are: (1) cystic disease with dilatation of the ducts, (2) epithelial changes, (3) stromal changes, (4) changes of both epithelium and stroma.

Cystic dilatation of the ducts is the most common change, and hence is responsible for the generic name given to this group of changes. It is also the change which is responsible for the majority of clinical and radiographic abnormalities. Multiple ducts are dilated and are usually filled with clear fluid, but may contain blood-stained fluid so as to produce the "blue-domed cyst of Bloodgood" (Fig. 2-1). Microscopically, the dilated ducts are usually lined by a flattened epithelium which is composed of the two types of cells normally found in the mammary duct, the myoepithelial cells which are located on the basement membrane and the more centrally located epithelial cells. In the fluid associated with the epithelial cells may be found lipid-laden macrophages, the so-called foam cells. The size of the ducts which are dilated varies from large subareolar ducts to small terminal ducts. Recognition of the dilatation of the terminal ducts is necessary so that this change may be distinguished from tubular carcinoma. The dilated ducts are frequently surrounded by dense fibrous tissue which may represent either compressed stroma or, when associated with inflammatory cells, scar tissue. There is wide variation in the degree of inflammatory cell infiltrate around dilated ducts, but it is rarely absent. This change has been emphasized with the term chronic cystic mastitis, which is frequently used interchangeably with cystic disease. Marked chronic inflammation with a predominance of plasma cells may occur in association with cystic disease. When it occurs in its absence, it is termed plasma cell mastitis. The tense, dilated cysts and the scar tissue around them are responsible for the hardness of some of these lesions.

Although the abnormality noted clinically may have been merely simple cysts or a variation in the density of the stroma, the surrounding breast tissue displays a remarkable range of alterations which are of more interest to the microscopist. Hyperplasia of the epithelium in the surrounding ducts is commonly seen. There is almost invariably hyperplasia of both the epithelial and myoepithelial cells—the hallmark of benign hyperplasia. The cellular hyperplasia may progress to the point where a simple lining can no longer

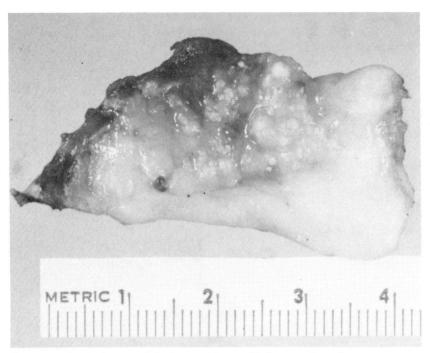

Fig. 2–1. Cystic disease of the breast. Note multiple cysts throughout the breast. These represent dilated ducts filled with fluid, or duct
ectasia. Gross × 2.5.

accommodate all of the cells, so that papillary foldings occur and the
ducts become distended. This is called papillomatosis (Fig. 2-2). An
alteration may occur in the type of cell participating in these
proliferating lesions, so that the cells develop eosinophilic granular
cytoplasm and large hyperchromatic nuclei, resembling those cells
seen in the apocrine sweat glands. Another example of proliferative
activity is seen in the breast that has undergone the physiologic
proliferation of lactation. In this situation, the epithelial cells
increase in size and number, filling the terminal ducts with distended vacuolated cytoplasm (Fig. 2-3). Occasionally a circumscribed area of the breast may continue to show this proliferative
change long into the post-partum period, after most of the breast has
returned to its resting state. This is the so-called lactating adenoma.
Atrophy of the epithelium may also occur and, occasionally, may
specifically suggest the microscopic appearance of a tubular carcinoma, from which it may be distinguished by the presence of both
cell types.

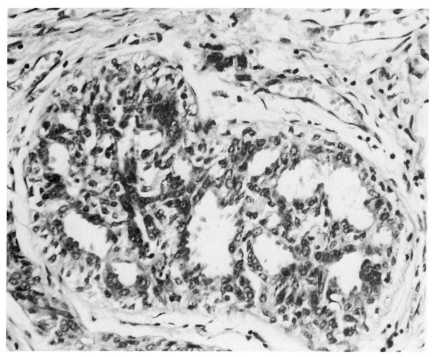

Fig. 2-2. Papillomatosis. An irregular proliferation of two types of cells inside the duct. The myoepithelial cells are evident adjacent to the basement membrane as cells with hyperchromatic round regular nuclei and clear cytoplasm. The epithelial cells line the lumens, are more columnar in shape, and have small projections into the lumens, at least in some areas. Their nuclei are polarized away from the luminal border. The nuclei vary from vesicular to reticular in chromatin pattern and are of different sizes. The irregular proliferation and the presence of both types of cells are the diagnostic features. Hematoxylin and eosin stain (H&E) × 300. Compare with Figure 2-9.

Isolated stromal changes may occur and may be focal in nature. When an increase in the connective tissue stroma of the breast occurs, it can produce a palpable abnormality (a fibrous mastopathy), which may be clinically suggestive of the induration produced by a malignant tumor. On histologic section the breast then shows an increase in the connective tissue stroma with little change in the epithelial elements.

Stromal and epithelial hyperplasia may occur together to produce two lesions, a circumscribed mass which is called a fibroadenoma, or a diffuse hyperplasia of both epithelial and stroma elements

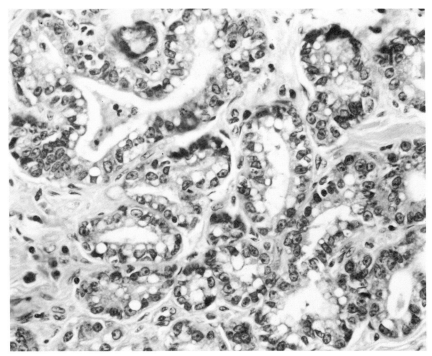

Fig. 2-3. Lactating breast. The ducts are lined by secreting columnar (epithelial) cells. Note the vacuoles of secretion on the luminal
side of the cell. The large vesicular nuclei with prominent nucleoli
are evidence of activity. The myoepithelial layer is not apparent.
H&E × 300.

called fibroadenosis. In the early states of either lesion, the fibroblasts in the stroma are markedly activated and produce abundant
collagen. Similarly, there is proliferation of the associated duct epithelium to produce the elongated slits characteristic of the lesion
(Fig. 2-4). These lesions are probably a localized response to estrogen, since they morphologically resemble both juvenile hypertrophy
and gynecomastia and are virtually never seen in an active stage
prior to puberty or after the menopause. As these lesions regress,
they may be seen in postmenopausal women as a collagenized lesion
which may be partially or almost completely calcified. This may
produce a truly rock-hard mass.

Another lesion in which both stromal and epithelial hyperplasia
are present is called sclerosing adenosis. Both gross and microscopic
appearances of this lesion may mimic carcinoma. Grossly the lesion
is firm, puckered and contains white flecks. Microscopically, the

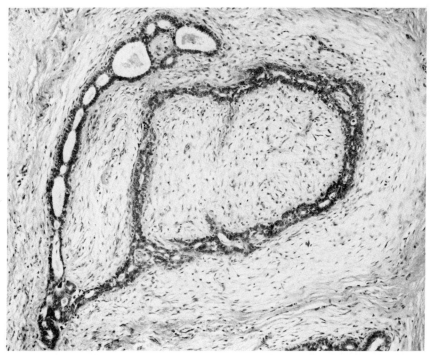

Fig. 2–4. Fibroadenoma. A proliferation of both stromal and epithelial elements. The elongated slit-like ducts are surrounded by a cellular stroma containing numerous proliferating fibroblasts. This pattern of fibroadenoma is termed intracanalicular and is associated with a rapidly enlarging lesion. H&E × 90.

lesions show varying degrees of proliferation of the epithelium of the terminal ducts which are distorted by surrounding scar tissue (Fig. 2–5). The major features which allow its recognition are its multicentricity, its lobular size, and its association with recognizable benign proliferative change in the lesion and in the adjacent breast tissue. Epithelial components of this lesion have been seen in perineural spaces (1) and in our laboratory we have seen benign breast tissue in axillary lymph nodes associated with sclerosing adenosis (2). Although epithelial cells within perineural spaces, or breast tissue within axillary lymph nodes, is usually associated with carcinoma, the natural history of this lesion is known to be benign. These lesions may contain focal areas of calcification, and thus be demonstrable on mammography.

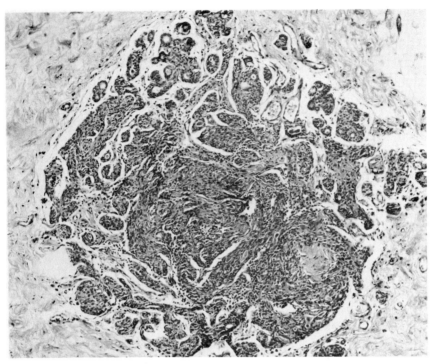

Fig. 2-5. Sclerosing adenosis. A proliferative sclerosing lesion which may be confused with carcinoma. It is the size of an expanded lobule, remnants of which are evident around the periphery. The irregular mass in the central portion is composed of proliferating epithelial and myoepithelial cells, basement membrane, fibrous tissue, and fibroblasts. Proliferation of the duct cells after the lobular architecture has been distorted by an inflammatory process is considered the genesis of this lesion. H&E × 90.

Intraductal Papilloma

Intraductal papillomas are regarded as benign tumors of the epithelium of large ducts. They are infrequently seen; we have seen ninety-one cases over a period of eighteen years (approximately one papilloma in 100 breast biopsies). They usually are associated with a serous or sanguineous nipple discharge, which may contain small papillary fragments of cells that are evident on cytologic examination. They are usually close to the areola, but may be found deeper in the breast and rarely are large enough to be palpable. Localization may require identification of the lesion by inserting a fine lachrymal probe into the bleeding duct.

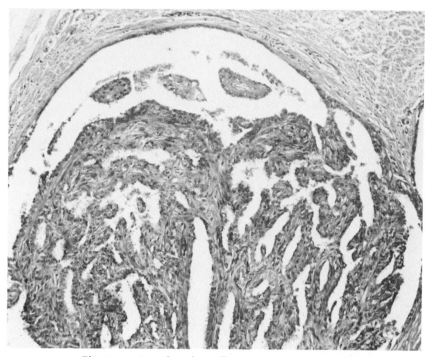

Fig. 2-6. Intraductal papilloma. The lesion is confined by a large duct which it distends. Although cellular, the lesion is essentially a set of branching fibrovascular stalks which are covered by a simple epithelium. Most of the lesion is seen in longitudinal section, but at the top, cross sections of the stalks are evident. A small vessel is evident in the center and the structure is covered by epithelium. H&E × 130.

Grossly, the papilloma is confined within the duct which has dilated to accommodate it. Microscopically, the lesion shows the proliferative changes of papillomatosis with which it may be associated in the surrounding breast. The majority of the lesions are readily recognizable as papillomas, benign neoplasms that are confined by the duct in which they arise. They arise from the wall of the duct as a fibrovascular stalk which is covered by hyperplastic epithelium that clearly shows both epithelial and myoepithelial hyperplasia (Fig. 2-6). In other lesions, however, the distinction from papillary carcinoma (which is subsequently discussed), is more difficult. The epithelial proliferation may become very striking and irregular, and the cells along the duct wall interact with the stroma in such a way as to produce pseudoinfiltration. Kraus and Neubecker have presented the differential features of papillary tumors of the breast, but these are useful only as a guide to the correct interpretation of the lesions (3). The obviously benign lesions can be readily recognized at the time of frozen section, and we are not reluctant to so diagnose those cases. We are, however, reluctant in some cases to distinguish between a proliferative papilloma and a papillary carcinoma on frozen section, and defer some of these cases until the entire lesion can be examined on paraffin sections.

Despite the morphologic similarity between intraductal papilloma and papillary carcinoma, there is no evidence to suggest that the papilloma progresses to papillary carcinoma (4, 5).

Papillary adenoma of the nipple is an even rarer lesion which represents a papillary lesion of the major ducts in the nipple itself. It presents as a mass in the nipple which may be ulcerated, clinically resembling Paget's disease. Microscopically, it shows an even greater tendency to pseudoinfiltration than does the intraductal papilloma and is therefore more readily confused with infiltrating carcinoma. Local resection is considered the treatment of choice.

Summary. Cystic disease with the varying types of proliferative components described above is quite common, although the percentage of women who develop it sometime during their life is not accurately known. The relationship of these changes to breast cancer is not clear. Gallagher and Martin (6) regard them as nonobligate preneoplastic lesions. Although it is unusual to see a breast cancer develop in the absence of microscopic evidence of cystic disease, certainly the great majority of patients with cystic disease do not develop breast cancer. Consequently, it is important to differentiate these changes from those described below under in situ carcinoma, which have a more significant relationship to invasive carcinoma.

In Situ Carcinoma

In situ or intraepithelial carcinoma of the breast is conceptually qualitatively different from the proliferative lesions discussed previously under cystic disease. In situ carcinoma is carcinoma which has not yet invaded the stroma and thus is *incapable* of spreading beyond the breast. It is one aspect of the minimal cancer concept noted below. In situ carcinoma is not detectable clinically. It is usually detected in the sections of the breast tissue which has been removed for some other reasons, usually the presence of a mass. It is therefore of utmost importance that the pathologist examine multiple sections of the breast biopsy which is received along with the clinically evident mass for which the biopsy was obtained. Removal of the lesion in the preinvasive stage results in cure of the patient without exception. The only qualification to the foregoing statement is that the surgeon and the pathologist must do what is necessary to assure themselves that the lesion is entirely noninvasive. To the surgeon, this challenge is a difficult one, since a small invasive carcinoma may go unnoticed. The pathologist must be certain that he has carefully examined all of the tissue which he has received and usually he will resort to subserial sectioning of the blocks in which in situ carcinoma has been found, as well as microscopic examination of any additional tissue which he might have recieved. Even after careful study, it is difficult to guarantee that invasion has not occurred.

In situ carcinoma in the breast is recognizable not so much from a difference in the individual cells, as is seen in other organs, but from a difference in the pattern which the cells form. It is divided into three categories on the basis of the types of patterns formed and the size of the ducts in which it occurs.

Paget's Disease. Paget's disease is a distinctive form of carcinoma of the breast first described by Sir James Paget in 1874 (10) and representing approximately 2 to 3 percent of all breast cancers. It is characterized by the accumulation of abnormal cells in the epidermis of the nipple in association with carcinoma in the underlying breast.

Both the exact nature of the characteristic cells in the epidermis and the method by which they arrive there remain subjects of dispute. The cells are large, generally round or oval, and have large vesicular nuclei, often with prominent nucleoli (Fig. 2-7). They may contain variable amounts of melanin, and at least some of the cells will usually show a positive reaction with one of the stains for mucopolysaccharides. The cells occur singly or in small groups, and mitotic figures are frequently present. These cells are regarded by most observers as carcinoma cells, and the most popular interpretation of the method by which they arrive in the epidermis is that they arise from an intraductal carcinoma of the breast and permeate through the epithelium of the collecting duct system to reach the overlying skin of the nipple. Since the associated underlying carcinoma is not infrequently multifocal in the breast, an alternative hypothesis is that these cells arise at the location in which they are

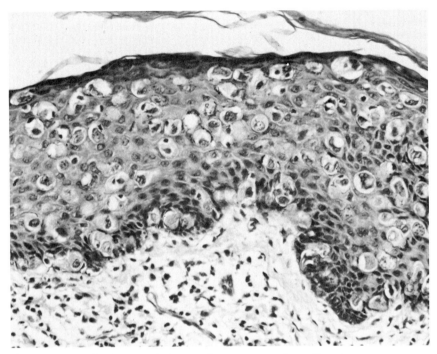

Fig. 2-7. Paget's disease of the nipple. Numerous large Paget's cells, occurring for the most part singly but also in small groups, are present throughout the epidermis of the nipple. The cytoplasm of the cells is pale or clear, and there is considerable nuclear pleomorphism. H&E × 270.

found, just as do the carcinoma cells of the other multiple foci within the breast.

Regardless of the precise nature of these cells or the mechanism by which they appear in the epidermis, their presence in the skin of the nipple is an indication of carcinoma of the breast. In our experience, and in that of most other observers, every well-studied case of Paget's disease of the nipple has contained intraductal and/or infiltrating carcinoma of the underlying breast (Fig. 2-8). The infiltrating carcinoma, if present, does not differ from breast carcinomas in general, nor do metastases, if they occur.

The progressive involvement of the nipple by the characteristic abnormal cells may produce visible and symptomatic changes of the nipple while the carcinoma is still intraductal, i.e., noninvasive, only. Since noninvasive carcinoma of the breast, in the absence of Paget's disease, is asymptomatic, this results in a significantly

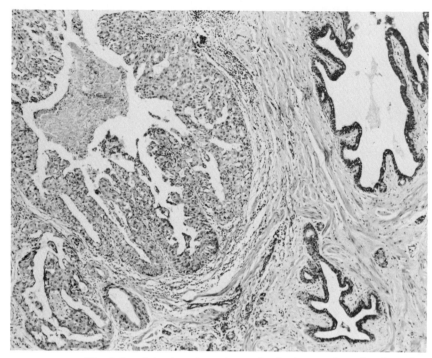

Fig. 2-8. Intraductal carcinoma in the large subareolar ducts beneath the nipple shown in Figure 2-7. Two uninvolved ducts are shown at the right. No invasive carcinoma was present in the breast. H&E × 70.

greater number of patients with Paget's disease receiving therapy while the tumor is noninvasive, and thus the overall survival of patients with this form of carcinoma is better than that of patients with breast cancer in general. It must be stressed that the improved prognosis of this group of patients rests entirely on the fact that a much higher percentage of them have noninvasive carcinoma only, for the invasive carcinoma associated with Paget's disease, with or without metastases, has essentially the same prognosis as does the corresponding stage of breast cancer in general. Thus, in the Memorial Hospital series, the net ten-year survival was 64 percent for Paget's disease, with 52 percent for duct carcinoma, reflecting the absence of invasive carcinoma in 17 percent of the former, but only 1 percent of the latter (11).

Intraductal Carcinoma. Intraductal carcinoma or in situ carcinoma in ducts is found in the larger ducts of the breast and generally

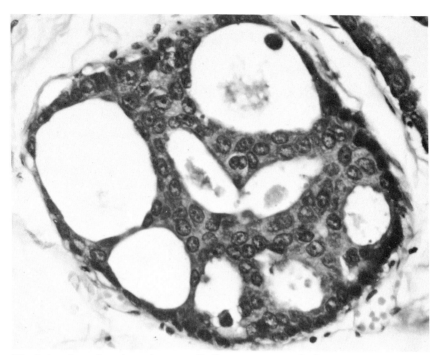

Fig. 2-9. Intraductal carcinoma, cribriform pattern. A fairly regular proliferation of cells in a small duct. Note that only one type of cell is evident in this proliferation and that the cells are less columnar in shape. The nuclei are large, but pleomorphism and anaplasia are not prominent. The diagnostic features are the regularity of the pattern and the lack of the normal two-cell population. H&E × 420. Compare this with Figure 2-2.

assumes one of four histologic patterns: cribriform, papillary, solid or comedocarcinoma. The cribriform pattern is one in which a proliferation of a single cell type occurs and forms a series of regular bridges of epithelium across the distended duct (Fig. 2-9). It is distinguished from the benign proliferative lesion by the presence of a single cell type and, paradoxically, by the regularity of the proliferation in the carcinoma and the irregularity of the proliferation in papillomatosis. The intraductal papillary carcinomas are those which will be described in the section on papillary carcinoma. The solid pattern is one in which a uniform population of cells fills and distends the large duct. The comedocarcinoma pattern essentially has the appearance of the solid pattern with necrosis of the centrally placed cells (Fig. 2-21).

Intraductal carcinoma is a lesion which is usually restricted in area and is associated with infiltrating carcinoma most of the time.

It is unusual to find intraductal carcinoma without finding associated infiltrating duct carcinoma, the ratio being approximately 1:20. The biologic significance of this observation is probably that intraductal carcinoma has a relatively brief preinvasive phase and is a virtually obligate precursor of invasive cancer. The practical significance of the observation is that identification of an invasive carcinoma must be diligently pursued by surgeon and pathologist alike.

Although intraductal carcinoma may extend into the terminal ducts of the lobule (and, similarly, in situ lobular carcinoma may extend from terminal ducts into the larger ducts), in situ lobular carcinoma is considered an entity separate from intraductal carcinoma.

In Situ Lobular Carcinoma. In situ lobular carcinoma is regarded as a lesion which is multifocal, often bilateral, and stays in the preinvasive phase for an extended period of time, sometimes for as much as twenty years. It is a relatively rare lesion; we see approximately ten cases a year in our laboratory (less than 10 percent of carcinomas). Because of the relative rarity of the lesion, the long duration of the in situ phase, and the understandable unwillingness of the surgeon to withhold therapy, relatively few untreated cases have been followed for as long as twenty years. McDivitt and his associates (7) reported a large series, fifty of these cases, from their experience at Memorial Hospital up until 1967. They found a cumulative actuarial risk of infiltrative carcinoma developing in the ipsilateral breast of 35 percent after twenty years, and in the contralateral breast a 25 percent incidence of in situ or invasive carcinoma after twenty years. Therefore, in situ lobular carcinoma is associated with invasive carcinoma far more frequently than are the proliferative changes seen in cystic disease. It is, however, associated with invasive carcinoma less frequently than intraductal carcinoma. We have recently seen a case which seems to sum up the significance of in situ lobular carcinoma. A woman in her midforties developed masses in both breasts and underwent bilateral breast biopsies five years ago. The masses in the breasts were found to be macrocysts. In the surrounding breast tissue, however, multifocal in situ lobular carcinoma was present in both breasts. For personal reasons, she chose not to have further treatment after the significance of the lesion had been explained to her. Recently, masses became palpable in both breasts again and bilateral breast biopsies were again performed. In one biopsy we were unable to

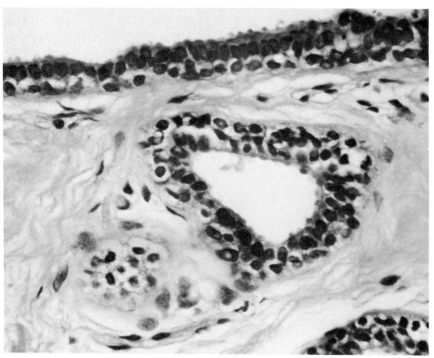

Fig. 2-10. Normal resting duct structure. Two ducts are present and both have the same histology. The larger duct at the top is lined by two layers of cells, the columnar epithelial cells on the luminal side and the clear myoepithelial cells adjacent to the basement membrane. Note that there is an apparent increase in the number of myoepithelial cells across the upper border of the smaller duct. H&E × 525.

find any evidence of in situ lobular carcinoma. This can be explained in one of three ways: the lesion had regressed, had been totally removed five years ago by biopsy, or the area in which the lesion was present was not biopsied. The last possibility seems most unlikely, since the disease had been quite diffuse and the second biopsy was a generous one. In the other breast, we found multifocal in situ and invasive lobular carcinoma.

In situ lobular carcinoma is present in the terminal ducts, which are the epithelial structures found in the lobules of the resting breast. As the lesion develops in these terminal ducts, the normal architecture (Fig. 2-10) (in which a central lumen is surrounded by a layer of epithelial cells and then a layer of clear myoepithelial cells inside the basement membrane) is effaced. The lumen of the duct

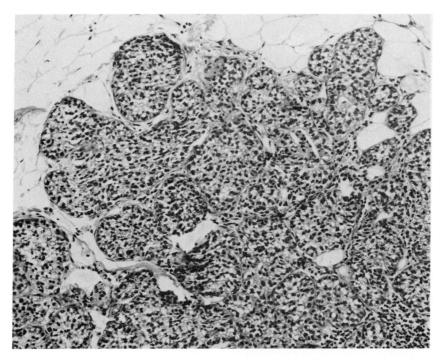

Fig. 2–11. In situ lobular carcinoma. In this lobule, the terminal ducts are distended by proliferating cells which have no recognizable orientation to each other. The lumens of most of the ducts are effaced. The cytoplasm of the cells is clear, and clear spaces are present in some of them. These clear spaces have been shown to represent intracellular lumens. The nuclei are hyperchromatic, but not significantly different from those seen in Figure 2–8. H&E × 160.

disappears and a single type of cell with a bland, round hyperchromatic nucleus and a small amount of eosinophilic cytoplasm fills and distends the duct (Fig. 2–11). Distinction between the epithelial and myoepithelial cell types is no longer possible. We have studied the lesion with the aid of the electron microscope and found features suggesting that the cell has some of the features of both epithelial and myoepithelial cell types in that intracytoplasmic lumina characteristic of the epithelial cell were present, as well as the myofibrillar material characteristic of the myoepithelial cell. The cells seemed sufficiently distinctive that we could distinguish them from the other types of breast cancer cells we studied (8). Lesser degrees of hyperplasia in the terminal ducts (Fig. 2–12) are not considered to have the same significance and have been designated blunt duct adenosis (9).

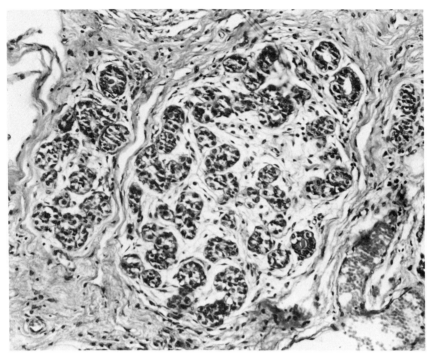

Fig. 2-12.   Blunt duct adenosis. Photomicrograph of a lobule showing the terminal ducts. Some of them (those in the upper right hand corner) are normal and comparable to the small ducts seen in Figure 2-10. In most of the others, the lumen is not apparent and there is a hyperplasia of the cells within the terminal ducts. The hyperplasia is relatively mild, however, and the ducts are not distended. Changes at this level are not of any known significance. H&E × 175. Compare this with Figure 2-11.

"Minimal Breast Cancer."   "Minimal breast cancer" is a term sometimes used to include very small scirrhous carcinomas, those histologic forms of carcinoma which have a more favorable prognosis and all forms of carcinoma which are in situ only. Although this type of terminology has some merit in drawing attention to the fact that all breast cancers are not identical and that a variety of factors may exert a favorable influence on the behavior of breast carcinoma in some patients, it tends to obscure the differences among the different types of cancer within this "group." It should be remembered that, unlike in situ carcinoma, all of the invasive carcinomas are capable of metastasizing and leading to the death of the patient, and that the prognosis noted below for certain types of invasive carcinoma is *relatively* more favorable than that for invasive breast cancer in general.

Invasive Carcinoma of the Breast. As noted above, all invasive carcinomas of the breast are capable of killing their host if untreated and given sufficient time to reach their endpoint. However, all those who have dealt with this disease extensively have been puzzled by the variation among breast carcinomas in their rate of progression to death. Therefore, rather than lump all of the carcinomas together, we will discuss in detail our system of subclassification of invasive carcinomas of the breast. The reason for subclassifying any group of neoplasms is to attempt to prognosticate the degree of biological aggressiveness from their histologic appearance. It must be remembered, however, that there is a high degree of overlap in the behavior of carcinomas among the groups and a disparity in the behavior among carcinomas in a given group. Histology is, therefore, only one consideration which the clinician must use to place the cancer on the continuum between earliest invasion and death of the patient from disseminated disease. Certain factors have been indentified which are of greater significance than the morphology of the carcinoma. Those patients with carcinoma in an advanced stage fare worse than those in which the lesion is in an early stage. Unfortunately, this is difficult to determine for some patients with a seemingly early cancer that may have disseminated metastases not discernible with even the most sophisticated techniques. The resistance of the host to the neoplasm is a factor which is probably of critical significance and yet is currently measurable only in the crudest of terms, the extent of spread of the cancer.

We will discuss the morphology of breast cancers in the following groups: (1) those which are generally less favorable, (2) those which are generally more favorable, (3) unusual carcinomas, and, (4) sarcomas. In addition, a histologic grading system applicable to all the carcinomas will be described. Unfortunately, the less favorable types comprise over 80 percent of breast cancer (see Table 2-1).

Cancers of the Breast with a Less Favorable Prognosis

Scirrhous Duct Carcinoma. This lesion comprises approximately 75 percent of the carcinomas of the breast and has a characteristic gross morphology.It is a hard mass, and this characteristic is responsible for the names which have been given to it, scirrhous (Greek *skirrhos*, hard) carcinoma, or carcinoma with productive fibrosis. The hardness of the lesion is the result of the desmoplastic reaction of the tissue of the breast. This is a proliferation of fibro-

Table 2–1.
Classification of Malignant Tumors of the Breast

In situ carcinoma	Paget's disease
	Intraductal carcinoma
	In situ lobular carcinoma
Invasive carcinoma	Scirrhous duct carcinoma
	Infiltrating lobular carcinoma
	Medullary carcinoma
	Colloid carcinoma
	Comedocarcinoma
	Papillary carcinoma
	Tubular carcinoma
	Metaplastic carcinoma
	Adenoid cystic carcinoma
	Childhood carcinomas
Sarcomas	Cystosarcoma phylloides
	Other sarcomas
Lymphomas	

blasts which are producing abundant collagen around the proliferating malignant epithelial cells. We are, therefore, denoting a characteristic of the host response to the neoplasm in our classification of this carcinoma. In the hard mass of fibrous tissue there are white or yellow streaks (Fig. 2–13). The proliferating carcinoma cells are present in three patterns. The designation duct carcinoma comes from the fact that frequently these invasive cells form small ducts (Fig. 2–14). However, they frequently do not differentiate into ducts, but grow in sheets or trabeculae (Fig. 2–15). They may exhibit growth in a single file between collagen fibrils so as to produce the so-called "Indian file" pattern (Fig. 2–16). These three patterns may be mixed. In addition, they frequently are associated with intraductal (or, occasionally, in situ lobular) carcinoma. The observation of in situ carcinoma in association with invasive carcinoma is, of course, the means by which in situ carcinoma was first recognized.

Statements regarding the epidemiology of carcinoma of the breast with no other specification (see Chapter 1) are generally referring to this type of carcinoma. The average age at which it is recognized is in the early fifties and the overall ten-year actuarial survival rate is approximately 50 percent. With carcinomas in Stage I (see Chapter 4) approximately 85 percent of the patients survive for five years. Patients with Stage II carcinomas have approximately a 66 percent five-year survival rate.

Discussions relating to the bilaterality of breast carcinoma generally refer to this type of carcinoma. Certainly they may be found bilaterally synchronously or metachronously, but one of the charac-

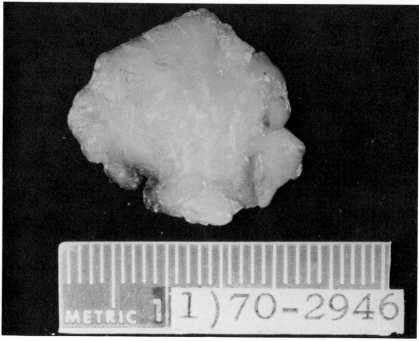

Fig. 2–13. Gross photograph of a typical infiltrating scirrhous duct carcinoma. The irregular border of the infiltrating carcinoma is evident. Coursing through the carcinoma are the characteristic chalky white streaks. × 3.

teristics necessary for the development of a subsequent new primary carcinoma is a sufficiently low level of biological aggressiveness, to allow most patients to live long enough for a second primary tumor to become manifest. Unfortunately, this is not a characteristic of this type of carcinoma.

Infiltrating Lobular Carcinoma. Infiltrating lobular carcinoma comprises about 7 percent of the carcinomas of the breast. It too is a firm tumor, but it does not have the hardness characteristic of the scirrhous duct carcinoma. Not infrequently, it is found multifocally in a breast and is found bilaterally, particularly synchronously, somewhat more commonly than is the duct carcinoma. It is the invasive carcinoma usually, although not exclusively, associated with in situ lobular carcinoma. Its histologic pattern is that of a carcinoma which is almost entirely in an "Indian file" pattern (Fig. 2–16), with the peculiar propensity to swirl around normal preexist-

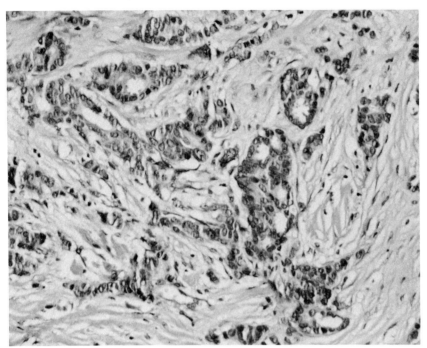

Fig. 2-14. Infiltrating scirrhous duct carcinoma. The dense collagen of the surrounding desmoplastic reaction is evident and is responsible for the firmness of the tumor. The cytoplasm of the infiltrating carcinoma cells is oriented around central lumens to form ducts. The nuclei are large and vesicular, and there is slight pleomorphism, but mitoses and bizarre nuclei are not present. H&E × 290.

ing ducts to form a target pattern (Fig. 2-17). Grossly, even though the tumor has an infiltrating border, its density is usually not such that it is readily distinguished and the microscopic appearance of the lesion may be difficult to separate from an inflammatory process, particularly on frozen section.

The distinction between scirrhous duct and infiltrating lobular carcinoma is not always a sharp one. Both may contain cells which are lined up in "Indian files." Intermediate types do exist. We restrict the diagnosis of infiltrating lobular carcinoma to those tumors which are comprised of small cells which are either individual or lined up in strands with a target pattern and prefer to see the in situ lobular carcinoma pattern associated with the invasive carcinoma. The cases which are ambiguous we classify as either scirrhous duct carcinomas (if that is the predominant pattern) or as infiltrating

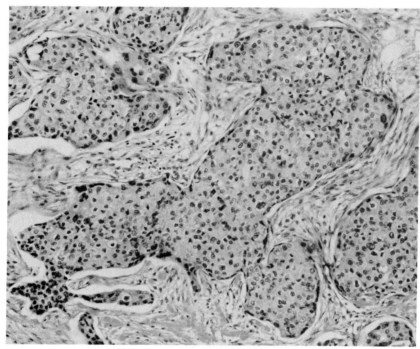

Fig. 2-15. Another infiltrating scirrhous carcinoma. The desmoplastic reaction is evident. Although the cells have considerably more cytoplasm than in the preceding figure, there is no orientation of the cells to form ducts. The nuclei are larger and considerably more pleomorphic, and mitotic figures are evident in at least three of the cells. H&E × 165.

breast carcinoma with features of both lobular and duct carcinoma. This is done to reserve the lobular carcinoma diagnosis for a cancer which has a heightened risk of bilaterality (12).

The survival figures for invasive lobular carcinoma with and without lymph node metastases are essentially the same as those for comparable scirrhous duct carcinomas; more than half the patients die of their disease in ten years (11). One peculiarity of the lymph node metastases of this cancer is that the small cells with scanty cytoplasm may form no pattern in the lymph node and evoke no desmoplastic response, so that the metastasis may histologically mimic a lymphoma (Fig. 2-18). This may lead to a difficult diagnostic problem if the cancer presents as an axillary metastasis without evidence of a primary tumor in the ipsilateral breast.

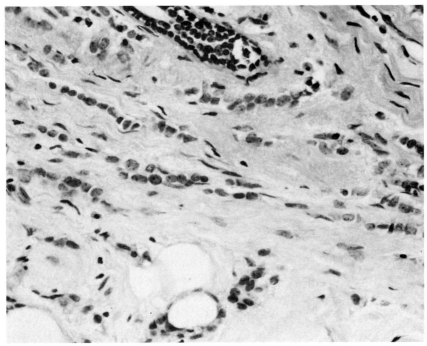

Fig. 2-16. "Indian-file" pattern. The cells of the carcinoma are small, have only a small amount of cytoplasm and hyperchromatic nuclei. The nuclei are molded by adjacent cells. This pattern is produced by the dense bundles of collagen which surround the cells. H&E × 390.

Types of Carcinoma with a Generally More Favorable Prognosis

A variety of types of carcinoma of the breast which can be readily identified histologically and which together comprise 10 to 15 percent of all breast cancer have a more favorable prognosis than scirrhous carcinoma. These are briefly described below.

Medullary Carcinoma. Medullary carcinoma consitutes approximately 5 percent of all breast cancer. Although it may be of any size, it is frequently a large bulky tumor when first seen by the physician, and hemorrhage and necrosis within the tumor are common. As a result, overlying skin changes such as erythema and even ulceration may occur, but these do not have the ominous prognostic significance of the skin changes in so-called "inflammatory carcinoma." On

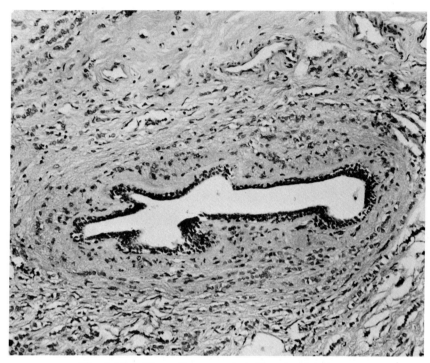

Fig. 2-17. "Target" pattern in infiltrating lobular carcinoma. The tumor cells infiltrate as single cells and as "Indian-files" in the layers of stroma around an uninvolved duct. H&E × 160.

the other hand, the tumors are characteristically circumscribed and are softer than scirrhous carcinoma, a combination of features which may lead to an erroneous clinical impression that the mass is benign, particularly if small.

Grossly, the tumors are circumscribed with a fleshy or firm consistency, sometimes cystic and often with areas of necrosis or hemorrhage. The dense fibrous tissue of scirrhous breast cancer is absent. Histologically, the tumor cells are large with abundant, finely granular cytoplasm and large nuclei, often with prominent nucleoli. There is very little cellular or nuclear pleomorphism, although scattered bizarre cells may be seen and mitoses are common. The cells occur in large sheets with little intervening stroma. A striking feature of most medullary carcinomas is a dense infiltrate of lymphocytes and/or plasma cells unrelated to areas of necrosis and uniformly present throughout the tumor (Fig. 2-19). This fea-

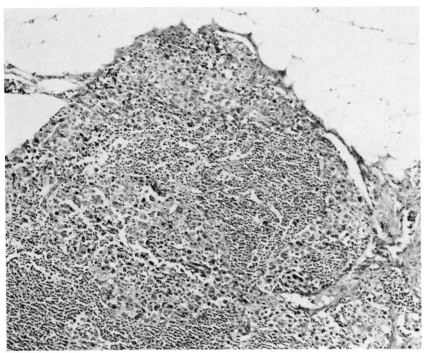

Fig. 2-18. Metastatic carcinoma in axillary lymph node. The cells of the carcinoma are growing in the peripheral sinus and sinusoids of the node. The lack of duct formation, large vesicular nuclei, and abundant eosinophilic cytoplasm present a histologic appearance which may be confused with a malignant lymphoma. H&E × 90.

ture, combined with the more favorable prognosis, obviously suggests a cellular defense mechanism against the tumor, but the precise mechanism and significance of the infiltrate is not known.

The definitely better prognosis of this type of cancer results both from the larger percentage of patients whose tumor has not metastasized and from the better survival in patients who have regional node metastasis. In the Memorial Hospital series, only 35 percent of these cases had regional metastases (vs. 54 percent for scirrhous carcinoma), and, of those that did, the net ten-year survival was 71 percent (vs. 52 percent) (11). An additional interesting observation is that, unlike breast cancer in general, very few deaths from carcinoma occurred in this group more than five years after mastectomy (9).

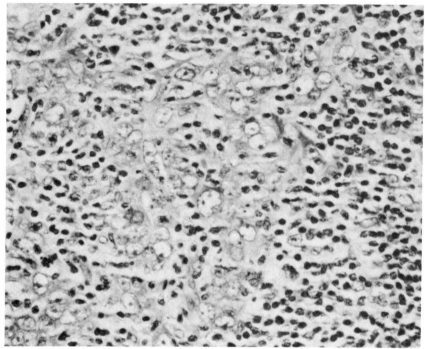

Fig. 2–19. Medullary carcinoma. A lymphocytic infiltrate is admixed with the characteristic large carcinoma cells having rather uniform vesicular nuclei and prominent nucleoli. Note the solid growth pattern, without duct formation, and the absence of a fibrous stromal response. H&E × 430.

Colloid (Mucinous) Carcinoma. The colloid or mucinous carcinoma constitutes 2 to 3 percent of breast cancer and in a disproportionate number of instances occurs in elderly patients. Like the medullary carcinoma, the tumor is usually circumscribed, softer than most cancers and not infrequently quite large. The excised tumor is usually sharply delineated, uniformly firm, and on sectioning has a gray glistening surface. Histologically, it consists of nests and acini of well-differentiated rather uniform small cells with small, dark nuclei and eosinophilic cytoplasm apparently floating in a sea of mucin (Fig. 2–20).

As stressed by Melamed and associates (13) and subsequently confirmed by others (14), the decidedly improved prognosis holds true for those patients whose tumors are largely or entirely of the appearance described above. Small mucinous areas may occur in ordinary breast cancer without altering the outlook, but, with

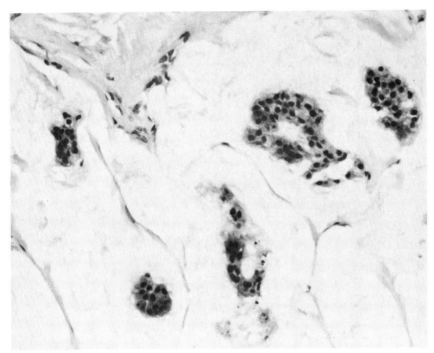

Fig. 2-20. Colloid (mucinous) carcinoma. Small apparently isolated clusters of rather bland-appearing cells lie in a pool of mucin. H&E × 270.

increasing relative amounts of this type of carcinoma, the prognosis improves. This improvement is the result solely of a lower incidence of lymph node metastasis, for, unlike medullary carcinoma, it is only those colloid carcinomas without such metastases that show a better survival than scirrhous duct carcinoma of a comparable stage. Thus, Melamed and his co-workers found an incidence of lymph node metastasis of 36 percent for pure colloid tumors and 47 percent for mixed patterns including a significant colloid component with five-year survival figures of 78 and 62.5 percent, respectively (13). The corresponding figures for those with only a slight colloid component are as bad or worse than those generally cited for breast cancer in general, as are those for any colloid carcinoma with axillary node metastases.

Comedocarcinoma with Infiltrating Carcinoma. The term comedocarcinoma refers to a pattern of intraductal carcinoma in which the growth is predominantly solid, but in which there is a prominent

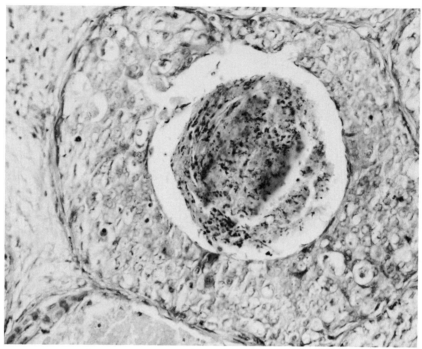

Fig. 2-21. Comedocarcinoma. Intraductal growth of tumor cells piled up several layers deep around the periphery. There is moderate pleomorphism of the cells and anaplasia of the nuclei. The characteristic feature is the necrosis of the cells in the center of the growth. H&E × 270.

amount of necrosis of the cells in the central areas of the ducts. The intraductal tumor may be extensive and involve an area several centimeters in diameter. Pressure on the excised tumor results in the expression of the necrotic material from the ducts, and it is this resemblance to a comedone that gives this particular type of tumor its name. The tumor cells are large, with hyperchromatic and pleomorphic nuclei, making recognition of this type of carcinoma generally quite simple (Fig. 2-21).

In some instances the tumor may be entirely confined to the ducts. However, it is not infrequently associated with areas of infiltrating carcinoma, generally of the ordinary scirrhous type. These areas may be multifocal within the lesion and are frequently quite small. In this situation, the tumor has a better prognosis than an infiltrating scirrhous duct carcinoma of comparable size. This appears to reflect merely the relatively small size of the infiltrating component compared to the relatively large amount of intraductal carcinoma.

Obviously, all gradations of these proportions may be seen, and only tumors which show only a small amount of infiltration should be included in this class. If this is done, it is seen that the incidence of axillary nodal metastasis is approximately half that of ordinary breast cancer, and the prognosis is similarly improved, with a crude five-year survival of 73 percent for this type of tumor, compared to 54 percent for infiltrating scirrhous duct carcinoma (9).

Papillary Carcinoma. Although papillary components can be found in a variety of types of breast cancer, the pure papillary carcinoma is an uncommon form, comprising 1 to 2 percent of all breast cancer.

The papillary carcinoma may be quite bulky and frequently is softer than the ordinary breast cancer, with a tendency to be circumscribed even if large. Central necrosis is common, and many of the tumors are frankly cystic. The infiltrating papillary carcinoma generally maintains a histologic pattern similar to papillary intraductal carcinoma, and the distinction between papillary carcinoma (Fig. 2-22) and benign papilloma (Fig. 2-6) may be difficult. Although general rules for recognizing each of the two lesions have been laid down and are for the most part valid (3, 9), there are sufficient exceptions to each of these guidelines that an attempt to concisely summarize them is apt to be more misleading than helpful. It can only be stressed that the accurate diagnosis of papillary carcinoma requires an experienced pathologist who is thoroughly familiar with the variations of both types of papillary breast disease.

Papillary carcinoma has a better prognosis at all clinical stages than does the scirrhous duct cancer (11). In addition, the incidence of nodal metastasis is much lower, with reported lymph node involvement less than one-third that of ordinary duct carcinoma and an overall crude five-year survival of 83 percent compared to 54 percent for duct carcinoma (9).

Tubular Carcinoma. The term tubular carcinoma refers to a very well-differentiated duct carcinoma of the breast, which is frequently smaller than the usual breast cancer. Grossly it resembles the common scirrhous duct carcinoma. Histologically it consists of well-differentiated cells forming orderly ducts and acini embedded in a scirrhous stroma. It may superficially resemble sclerosing adenosis, but the lumens of the ducts tend to remain patent rather than compressed by the stroma, and frequently only a single layer of epithelium is present instead of the usual double layer (Fig. 2-23). It thus represents the extremely well-differentiated aspect of the

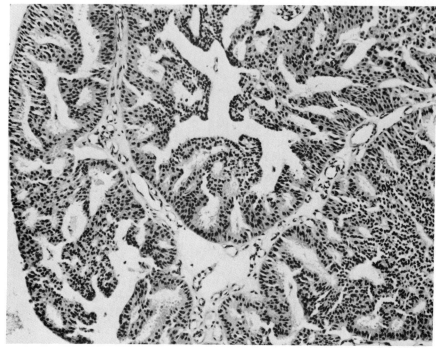

Fig. 2-22. Papillary carcinoma. Compare with the intraductal papilloma (Fig. 2-6), taken at the same magnification. The carcinoma shows papillary and interlacing groups of epithelial cells unsupported by fibrovascular stalks. The cells are of one type and relatively uniform, unlike the admixture of cell types seen in the benign lesion. H&E × 130.

histologic grading system described below, and it is apparently on this basis and the frequent small size of the lesion that the more favorable prognosis rests.

Since tubular carcinomas merely represent the best differentiated examples of a spectrum of tumors, meaningful incidence figures are difficult to obtain and will vary with the strictness of the diagnostic criteria. There is no question, however, that lymph node metastases are less frequent and patient survival better with this type of tumor than with breast cancer in general (15).

Histologic Grading of Breast Cancer

Bloom and his associates have used a system for defining the cellular characteristics of breast carcinomas in order to prognos-

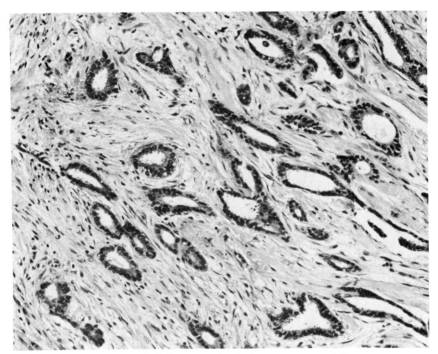

Fig. 2-23. The very well differentiated tubular carcinoma of the breast, which must be distinguished from sclerosing adenosis. Note the absence of two-cell types, the patent lumina, and the desmoplastic nature of the stroma. Compare with Figure 2-5. H&E × 205.

ticate the degree of biological aggressiveness, or the rate at which the tumor is developing in the breast. The cells of the carcinoma are examined for three characteristics: their ability to form ducts, the pleomorphism of their nuclei, and the mitotic rate. From one to three points are assigned in each category. Those tumors with well-marked duct formation are assigned one point, and those with little or no duct formation are assigned three points. Those with fairly uniform nuclei resembling those of normal cells are assigned one point, and those with bizarre nuclei which vary considerably are assigned three points. Those with a low mitotic rate are assigned one point, and those with a high mitotic rate are assigned three points. The points are totaled and the carcinomas are assigned to Grade I if the total is 3, 4, or 5; Grade II if the total is 6 or 7; and Grade III if the total is 8 or 9. On the average, the prognosis of the Grade III cancers is approximately half as good as that of the Grade I carcinomas in the opinion of the authors (16).

To an extent, this system parallels the categories previously described in that the tubular, papillary, and colloid carcinomas, which we have considered relatively favorable histologic types, fit into the Grade I category because of their formation of ducts or papillae and low mitotic rate. The lobular carcinoma, however, would fit into the Grade II category because of its lack of duct formation and low mitotic rate. As noted earlier, this pattern has been correlated with a relatively poor prognosis. Also, the medullary carcinoma, which is considered a relatively favorable cell type by all observers, would be classed as a Grade III carcinoma, since it does not form ducts, has pleomorphic nuclei, and a high mitotic rate. The paradoxical behavior of the medullary carcinoma has been noted by Bloom and associates.

The value of the system may be in its application to the largest group of carcinomas, which we have designated scirrhous duct carcinoma, in separating them into three groups. Other criteria have been offered to separate this large group of cancers into more or less favorable lesions. Among them are the character of the infiltrative border (17), the stellate and knobby configuration (6), and the presence of noninvasive carcinoma (18).

Unusual Forms of Cancer

In addition to the types of carcinoma discussed above, there are tumors of the breast which represent either very unusual forms of carcinoma or malignant tumors not of epithelial origin. These tumors are briefly considered below.

Metaplastic Carcinoma. Very infrequently a carcinoma of the breast may contain areas in which the differentiation of the cells is distinctly different from what one would anticipate in breast tissue. Frequently these are spindle-shaped cells without other distinguishing features, but there may be either unusual epithelial types, such as squamous cells (Fig. 2–24), or nonepithelial differentiation to osteoid or cartilage (Fig. 2–25). In tumors in which an element of characteristic breast cancer is present, these unusual areas are interpreted as metaplastic changes of the malignant epithelial cells.

The largest single series of such tumors (forty patients) has been reviewed by Huvos and his associates (19), who divided them into two groups. One group of twenty-four patients whose tumors had spindle and squamous metaplasia showed an incidence of lymph node metastasis (54 percent) and five-year survival (65 percent)

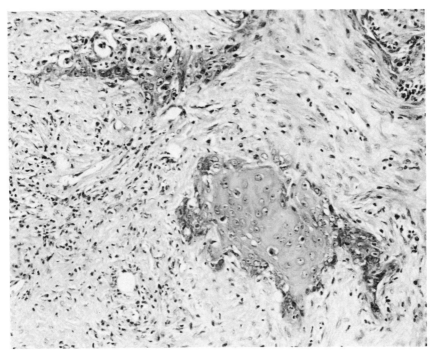

Fig. 2-24. Squamous metaplasia in mammary carcinoma. A portion of the focus of carcinoma in the upper left resembles a more ordinary pattern of breast carcinoma, while that near the center shows squamous differentiation. H&E × 165

similar to breast carcinoma in general. The second group of 16 patients, with osseous and cartilaginous metaplasia, had a lower incidence of node metastases (19 percent) but also a lower five-year survival (38 percent), suggesting that these tumors metastasize to a greater degree by the bloodstream.

Adenoid Cystic Carcinoma. The adenoid cystic carcinoma is a truly rare form of breast cancer, and we are aware of only fifty-six reported cases. Ths histologic appearance is identical to that of the adenoid cystic carcinoma of the salivary gland and must be differentiated from the cribriform pattern of scirrhous carcinoma (Fig. 2-26).

Metastasis from this tumor is extremely unusual, and only two deaths, each involving pulmonary metastases, have been reported (20, 21). Local recurrences have been seen, but with these two exceptions have been successfully treated (22). It is noteworthy that no axillary lymph node metastases have been reported.

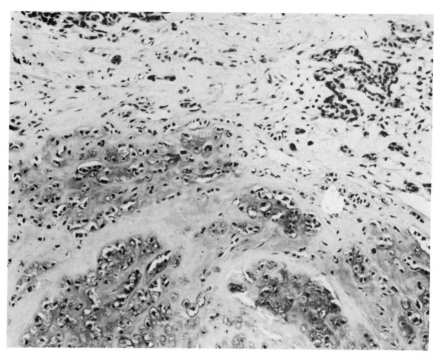

Fig. 2-25. Cartilaginous metaplasia. The tumor in the upper right shows the epithelial characteristics of a carcinoma, with a narrow transitional zone leading to the tumor in the lower portion showing chondroid differentiation. H&E × 140.

Cystosarcoma Phyllodes.   The cystosarcoma is a tumor of the breast which in many ways resembles a fibroadenoma, with both an epithelial and a nonepithelial component generally arranged in the same fashion as in that tumor. Like the fibroadenoma, it occurs only in females. In spite of the ominous name, the majority of these tumors are benign.

Grossly the tumor resembles the fibroadenoma, but frequently has a less regular margin, which may in some instances be clearly less distinct. However, the recognition of the cystosarcoma rests on its histologic appearance. The stroma is invariably more cellular than that of the fibroadenoma and is composed of fibrous or spindle cells with a variable degree of myxomatous change (Fig. 2-27). The epithelium usually shows varying degrees of hyperplasia and atypia, but a frankly malignant epithelial component (carcinoma) is extremely rare.

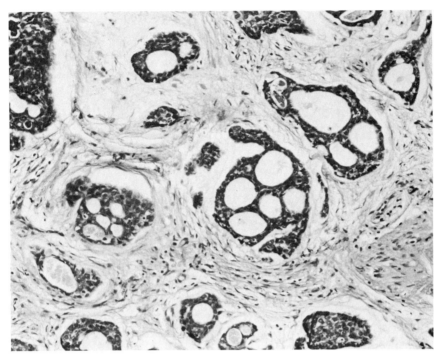

Fig. 2-26.   Adenoid cystic carcinoma of the breast. This rare pattern
of breast carcinoma must be distinguished from the more common
cribriform pattern of intraductal carcinoma (Fig. 2-7). H&E × 160.

The distinction between benign and malignant cystosarcoma may
be quite difficult and is based on the microscopic appearance of the
stroma. In a detailed study of ninety-four patients, Norris and
Taylor (23) found infiltrative margins, cellular atypia and frequent
mitoses were the most reliable indices of malignancy, particularly
when occurring in combination (Fig. 2-28). Since these features may
vary within the same tumor, thorough sampling is necessary, but
even after careful evaluation it may be impossible to guarantee that a
cystosarcoma will not prove to be malignant. In the series noted,
recurrences occurred in 30 percent of the patients, and 17 percent
died of metastatic tumor, which involves the lungs and other distant
sites and very rarely involves axillary lymph nodes.

Sarcomas and Lymphomas.   The breast may rarely be the site of
primary soft-tissue sarcomas and lymphomas similar to those that
occur elsewhere in the body.

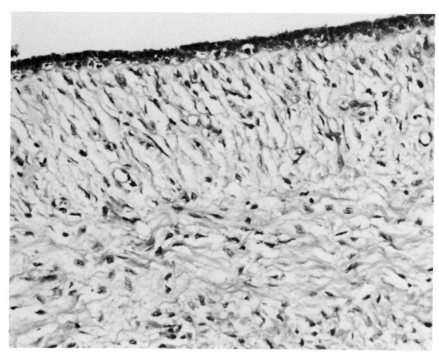

Fig. 2-27. A histologically benign cystosarcoma phyllodes, showing the well-differentiated and orderly pattern of the stroma. The epithelium of a large duct-like space is shown at the top. Compare with Figure 2-28. H&E × 275.

A wide variety of types of sarcoma have been reported. The prognosis appears to be in general related to the degree of differentiation, with well over half the patients surviving more than five years (24). One notable exception is the angiosarcoma (Fig. 2-29), which is almost always a rapidly fatal tumor, although one patient treated in this hospital is living free of disease ten years after mastectomy. Metastasis to axillary lymph nodes from an angiosarcoma of the breast has not been reported, and lymph node metastasis from any sarcoma of the breast is extremely rare.

Lymphomas may occur as isolated tumors of the breast (Fig. 2-30), but the patient should be carefully evaluated to exclude more generalized lymphoma presenting in this fashion. Similarly, it should be recalled that the much more common medullary carcinoma may be difficult to distinguish from lymphoma.

Breast Carcinoma in the Male. Only 1 percent or less of carcinoma of the breast occurs in male patients. It generally presents as a

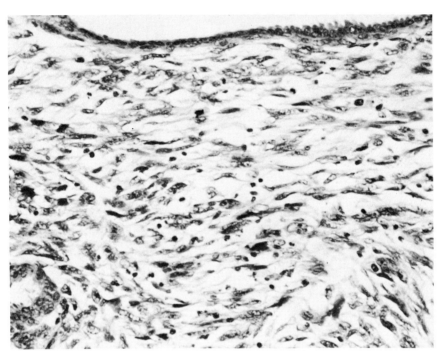

Fig. 2–28. A malignant cystosarcoma which subsequently metastasized. The stromal cells have pleomorphic, often hyperchromatic nuclei, and a mitotic figure is present above the center of the field. The epithelium at the top is not atypical. Compare with Figure 2–27. H&E × 275.

mass in the breast and, due to the relatively small amount of breast tissue in the male, will in almost all instances be found beneath the areola or in close proximity to it. For the same reason, fixation to the skin or underlying tissue is common, as is nipple discharge. The histologic appearance of the tumors is similar to the variety of types seen in the female breast, including Paget's disease, although in situ lobular carcinoma is notably not seen. It appears that the favorable histologic types of cancer in the female have a better prognosis in the male also (25).

Carcinoma in Children. In addition to the forms of carcinoma already described, McDivitt and Stewart reported a series of seven cases of a distinctive form of cancer in young children (26). Grossly similar to other carcinomas, the tumor shows an infiltrating pattern of large cells with clear or pale cytoplasm and PAS-positive secretory material within the cells and in small duct-like spaces (Fig.

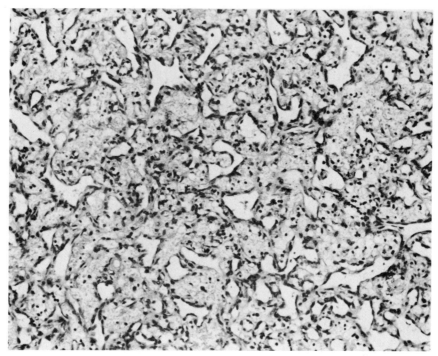

Fig. 2-29. Angiosarcoma of the breast. In spite of the lack of anaplastic features, these tumors have a very poor prognosis. H&E × 175.

2-31). No metastases were seen in their cases, but in a subsequent report a similar tumor showed a single lymph node metastasis (27). Recurrence following local excision has been reported (26), but we are unaware of the death of any patient resulting from this type of cancer.

Carcinoma of the breast of the more usual types is also extremely rare in young girls, and the very few cases of the usual types of carcinoma that have been reported have been almost entirely in patients in the second decade. We have seen only one such patient at this hospital, a sixteen-year-old girl who died fourteen months after mastectomy from a large in situ and infiltrating lobular carcinoma with extensive metastases.

Mastectomy Specimen

Study of the mastectomy specimen in the surgical pathology laboratory is carried out to provide information of prognostic sig-

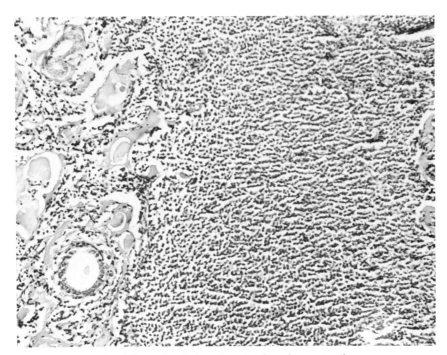

Fig. 2-30. Poorly differentiated lymphocytic lymphoma in the breast. Sheets of tumor cells have infiltrated and largely replaced the breast architecture, remnants of which are seen on the left. H&E × 190.

nificance for the patient and to study the disease process and its therapy.

The specimen is examined for residual tumor in order to determine the extent of the tumor and the histologic type, both of which are of prognostic significance as discussed above. These may be more readily apparent after examination of the entire lesion than after examination of a biopsy which is less than excisional. Staging is also aided by the microscopic demonstration of the relationship of the cancer to the skin and to the fascia, if these are available. Permeation of the dermal lymphatics by tumor cells is a very grave sign. Demonstration of vascular invasion in the breast is of prognostic significance, but correlates almost uniformly with the presence of axillary lymph node metastases. Therefore its prognostic significance is that of the metastatic disease. Its value lies in predicting the presence of axillary node metastases if lymphadenectomy was not performed.

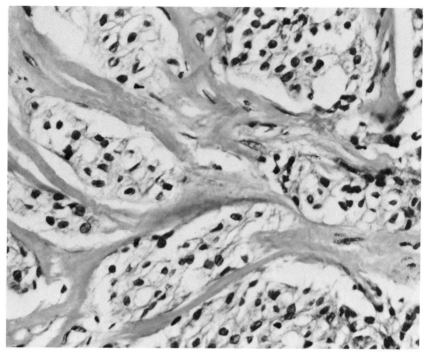

Fig. 2-31. The rare carcinoma of the breast in young children, showing the characteristic large cells with pale or clear cytoplasm infiltrating the dense stroma. H&E × 390.

If a lymphadenectomy has been performed, this must be thoroughly examined, since it provides information of the greatest prognostic significance. It is important that all the nodes be examined microscopically. In Chapter 4 we note that the clinical impression of axillary lymph nodes is incorrect in 30 percent of the cases, i.e., 30 percent of patients thought to have negative nodes are shown to have metastases microscopically, and, similarly, 30 percent of patients with enlarged lymph nodes are shown to have reactive hyperplasia rather than metastatic disease. Not only the presence of lymph node metastases but also the number of lymph node metastases are of significance. Those patients with one to three axillary lymph nodes containing metastatic tumor have a considerably better prognosis than those patients with four or more axillary lymph nodes containing metastatic tumor (see Chapter 4). In patients with subareolar or inner quadrant lesions, the presence of axillary lymph node metastases correlates with the presence of internal mammary lymph node metastases in about 60 percent of the cases, while internal mammary node metastases are found in only 15 percent of those patients whose axillary nodes are free of tumor (25). Extension of metastatic carcinoma from the lymph node into the axillary adipose tissue is correlated with a graver prognosis than the presence of metastatic disease confined to the lymph node (9). In addition, the noninvolved axillary lymph nodes have been studied for an indication of the host response to the carcinoma. The presence and degree of sinus histiocytosis (proliferation of histiocytes in the sinusoids of the lymph nodes) has been proposed as an indication of the effectiveness of the host response. Numerous authors have written on this topic in an attempt to correlate the degree of sinus histiocytosis with both the inflammatory cell infiltrate around the primary tumor and the ultimate survival rate. However, the evidence does not clearly indicate that sinus histiocytosis is evidence of an effective response by the host against the tumor.

Examination of the mastectomy specimen can also provide information regarding the nature of the disease and appropriate therapy. Shah et al. (28) studied over 500 patients who underwent mastectomy after apparent excisional biopsy and found residual carcinoma in 59 percent of the mastectomy specimens. Residual cancer was found most commonly, interestingly enough, in those patients with very small carcinomas and those with tumors larger than 4 cm, and somewhat less frequently in patients with carcinomas 1 to 4 cm in diameter. This held true for all histologic types of carcinoma seen. These authors did not address the problem of the quadrant of the breast in which the residual carcinoma was found. However, Qualheim and Gall (29) and Tellem et al. (30) have studied mastectomy specimens with large sections and have found carcinoma in quadrants of the breast unconnected to the grossly visualized tumor in 37 percent and 26 percent respectively. From studies such as these, it seems clear that carcinoma of the breast is a more diffuse disease process than that suggested by the clinical or gross pathologic examination of the palpable lesion.

Examination of the mastectomy specimen has also been of great value to the pathologist's attempts to segregate the proliferative changes in the duct epithelium which are associated with carcinoma from those which are not. As mentioned above, in situ carcinoma was identified from the study of cancer-bearing mastectomy specimens by its association with invasive carcinoma.

Metastatic Carcinoma of the Breast

Like other carcinomas, those of the breast metastasize both by lymphatics and by the bloodstream. The primary lymphatic drainage is to the ipsilateral axillary nodes and much of the discussion regarding the appropriate initial therapy of breast cancer involves the treatment directed at these nodes. Less widely appreciated is the fact that, for lesions located medially in the breast, the internal mammary nodes are involved as frequently as are the axillary nodes, and for all breast cancers these nodes are involved in approximately one-third of the patients (9). Valuable prognostic information is obtained from a mastectomy specimen by determining the exact number of axillary nodes involved by metastases. Additional information can be derived by dividing the axillary contents into levels, conventionally designating the nodes beneath the pectoralis minor muscle as level II, and the areas lateral and medial to the muscle levels I & II, respectively. This is difficult to do accurately, however, unless these levels are marked by the surgeon during the resection and cannot be done for those operations in which the pectoralis muscles are not removed.

Breast cancers may metastasize widely and unpredictably, and these metastases may first become obvious only after an apparent disease-free interval of many years. Metastatic breast cancer is notorious for its variable appearance and may on occasion mimic other lesions, e.g., lymphomas, and this should be taken into consideration when evaluating any tissue from a patient who has had a carcinoma of the breast. Unlike other carcinomas which not infrequently have "silent" primary tumors, carcinoma of the breast rarely presents clinically as a metastatic lesion in the absence of an easily detectable primary tumor. On the few occasions when this occurs, the metastasis is usually in an axillary lymph node on the same side as the occult primary tumor.

References

1. Taylor, H. B., and Norris, H. J. 1967. Epithelial invasion of nerves in benign diseases of the breast. *Cancer* 20:2245.
2. Edlow, D. W., and Carter, D. 1973. Heterotopic epithelium in axillary lymph nodes. *Am. J. Clin. Path.* 59:666.
3. Kraus, F. T., and Neubecker, R. D. 1962. The differential diagnosis of papillary tumors of the breast. *Cancer* 15:444.
4. McDivitt, R. W., Holleb, A. I., and Foote, F. W., Jr. 1968. Prior breast disease in patients treated for papillary carcinomas. *Arch. Path.* 85:117.

5. Pellettiere, E. V. 1971. II: Clinical and pathological aspects of papillomatous disease of the breast: Follow-up study of 97 patients treated by local excision. *Am. J. Clin. Path.* 55:740.
6. Gallagher, H. S., and Martin, J. E. 1969. Early phases in the development of breast cancer. *Cancer* 24:1170.
7. McDivitt, R. W., Hutter, R. V. P., Foote, F. W., Jr., and Stewart, F. W. 1967. In situ lobular carcinoma: A prospective follow-up study indicating cumulative patient risks. *JAMA* 201:82.
8. Carter, D., Yardley, J. H., and Shelley, W. M. 1969. Lobular carcinoma of the breast. An ultrastructural comparison with certain duct carcinomas and benign lesions. *J. Hopkins Med. J.* 125:25.
9. McDivitt, R. W., Stewart, F. W., and Berg, J. W. 1967. Tumors of the breast. *Atlas of Tumor-Pathology.* Second Series. Fascicle 2. A.F.I.P.
10. Paget, J. 1874. Disease of the mammary areola preceding cancer of the mammary gland. *St. Barth. Hosp. Rep.* 10:87.
11. Berg, J. W., Schottenfeld, D., Hutter, R. V. P., and Foote, F. W., Jr. 1969. Histology, epidermiology and end results: The Memorial Hospital Cancer Registry. U.S.A.
12. Fechner, R. E. 1972. Infiltrating lobular carcinoma. *Cancer* 29:1539.
13. Melamed, M. R., Robbins, G. F., and Foote, F. W., Jr. 1961. Prognostic significance of gelatinous mammary carcinoma. *Cancer* 14:669.
14. Norris, H. J., and Taylor, H. B. 1965. Prognosis of mucinous (gelatinous) carcinoma of the breast. *Cancer* 18:879.
15. Taylor, H. B., and Norris, H. J. 1970. Well-differentiated carcinoma of the breast. *Cancer* 25:689.
16. Bloom, H. J. G., and Richardson, W. W. 1957. Histologic grading and prognosis in breast cancer: A study of 1409 cases of which 359 have been followed for 15 years. *Brit. J. Cancer* 11:359.
17. Kouchoukos, N. T., Ackerman, L. V., and Butcher, H. R., Jr. 1967. Prediction of axillary nodal metastases from the morphology of primary mammary carcinomas. *Cancer* 20:948.
18. Silverberg, S. G., and Chitale, A. R. 1973. Assessment of significance of proportion of intraductal and infiltrating tumor growth in ductal carcinoma of the breast. *Cancer* 32:830.
19. Huvos, A. G., Lucas, J. C., and Foote, F. W., Jr. 1973. Metaplastic breast carcinoma. Rare form of mammary cancer. *N.Y. State J. Med.* 73:1078.
20. Nayer, H. R. 1957. Cylindroma of the breast with pulmonary metastasis. *Dis. Chest* 31:324.
21. O'Kell, R. T. 1964. Adenoid cystic carcinoma of the breast. *Missouri Med.* 61:855.
22. Cavanzo, F. J., and Taylor, H. B. 1969. Adenoid cystic carcinoma of the breast. *Cancer* 24:740.
23. Norris, H. J., and Taylor, H. B. 1967. Relationship of histologic features to behavior of cystosarcoma phyllodes. *Cancer* 20:2090.
24. Norris, H. J., and Taylor, H. B. 1968. Sarcomas and related mesenchymal tumors of the breast. *Cancer* 22:22.
25. Haagensen, C. D. 1971. *Diseases of the breast.* Second edition. Philadelphia: W. B. Saunders Company.
26. McDivitt, R. W., and Stewart, F. W. 1966. Breast carcinoma in children. *JAMA* 195:388.
27. Byrne, M. P., Fahey, M. M., and Gooselaw, J. G. 1973. Breast cancer with axillary metastases in an eight and one-half year old girl. *Cancer* 31:726.
28. Shah, J. P., Rosen, P. P., and Robbins, G. F. 1973. Pitfalls of local excision in the treatment of carcinoma of the breast. *Surg., Gynec. & Obstet.* 136:721.
29. Qualheim, R. E., and Gall, E. A. 1957. Breast cancer with multiple sites of origin. *Cancer* 10:460.
30. Tellem, M., Prive, L., and Meranze, D. R. 1962. Four quadrant study of breasts removed for carcinoma. *Cancer* 15:10.

3. THE ROLE OF RADIOLOGICAL EXAMINATIONS IN THE MANAGEMENT OF PATIENTS WITH SUSPECTED BREAST CANCER

Atsuko Heshiki and Floyd Osterman, Jr.

In recent years, the use of radiological procedures to detect early breast cancer has increased markedly. Five-year mortality has been reduced by the use of both repetitive clinical examinations and radiographic imaging of the breast (mammography) (13). In addition to conventional film and low-dose film mammography, xeroradiography has been widely employed in the imaging of the soft tissues, including the breast. Radiographic contrast may also be injected into the ductal system of the breast as an additional technical maneuver. Another procedure in wide use is thermography, which employs infra-red photography rather than X-ray imaging. The use of computerized tomographic scanning and diagnostic ultrasound are now being employed in mammographic imaging; however, the utility of these two relatively new procedures has yet to be demonstrated in the early detection of breast neoplasia.

In the following discussion, conventional film and low-dose film mammography, xeromammography, mammary duct injection, and thermography are briefly described and the description of each procedure is correlated with their respective advantages and disadvantages. The indications for these procedures are also briefly discussed.

Conventional Film Mammography

Mammography was developed and popularized by Gershon-Cohn (4), Leborgne (7), and Egan (3). This examination can be performed in most hospitals and many radiology offices by modifying the usual X-ray equipment with the addition of a Molybdenum target X-ray tube to provide low-intensity, high-contrast technique. Using a light-proof packet containing fine-grain film, cephalo-caudad and lateral views of the breast are obtained. The radiographies of the breast enable one to see many of the internal structures, but small lesions may be difficult to detect or fully characterize, particularly in a dense fibrous breast. Conventional film mammography is effective in detecting lesions in women whose breasts have extensive fatty infiltration. Compared to low-dose mammography and xeroradiography, the exposure time for conventional mammography is quite long, generally in the order of two to six seconds, consequently, conventional mammography delivers significant amounts of irradiation to the patient. Although adjacent and deep structures receive little irradiation because the X-ray beam employed is of low energy and does not penetrate deeply, the breast does receive a significant dose of irradiation; Gilbertson (5) has calculated that each breast receives three to four roentgens per view on the inner surface.

Low-Dose Mammography

Low-dose mammography (12) is accomplished by a radiographic technique which is similar to conventional mammography. This procedure employs a single-emulsion radiographic film held in intimate contact with a single high-detail intensifying screen which reduces image blurring associated with standard double emulsion film, but provides more contrast than nonscreen conventional mammographic film. The radiation dose is one-sixth to one-tenth that of conventional mammography due to the intensifying screen. A disadvantage of low-dose mammography is that calcific densities within the breast may be confused with tiny artifacts caused by dust particles. These artifacts may occur whenever intensifying screens are used and occasionally necessitate a repeat exposure.

Xeroradiography

Xeroradiography of the breast was developed and popularized by Wolfe (15) and Martin (9). A standard X-ray generator is used as the radiation source in xeroradiography, but the radiographic image is recorded xerographically rather than photographically (2, 15). X-rays are absorbed in a thin photoconductive layer of Selenium (Se) which has been precharged to a high-positive electrostatic potential. In the immediate area of an X-ray interaction, the conductivity of the Se layer is momentarily increased and a fraction of the electrostatic potential discharges. The information in a transmitted beam is thereby recorded in the surface charge remaining on the Se plate. Areas with little remaining surface charge correspond to high X-ray intensity—for example, areas of fat in the breast. Conversely, areas with high remaining surface charge correspond to low X-ray intensity or high object density, such as a tumor mass or bone.

The surface-charge image is visualized by exposing the Se layer to an aerosol of fine blue-charged particles (toner). Areas of high-charge density on the selenium plate accumulate proportionately greater amounts of blue toner than areas of lower-charge density. Therefore, areas of high object density, such as a tumor mass, appear dark on the powder image in contrast to lighter shades of blue below areas of low object density. The powder image on the selenium plate is transferred and fused to plastic-coated paper for interpretation and storage.

The xeroradiographic print has excellent resolution and accentuates structural differences by "edge enhancement." The process of edge enhancement refers to the build-up of the blue toner particles on the image print corresponding to areas of abrupt change in density in the radiographed object. Thus small tumor microcalcifications are easily detected, due to enhancement of the particle border. The thicker and thinner portions of the breast are satisfactorily exposed on the same print, due to the wide exposure latitude afforded by xeroradiography. Therefore, the dense stromal pattern as well as the skin line can be seen on the same print. The radiation dosage to the patient is also significantly less than conventional film mammography.

Although opinion is divided among radiologists as to whether film mammography or xeroradiography is more accurate, the editor, Dr. Baker, feels that, at least for the surgeon or physician without special training in radiology, xeroradiography is a better technique. The xeroradiographic films are easier to interpret compared to mammographic films. Furthermore, xeroradiography of a biopsy specimen provides more accurate localization of a clinically occult lesion than does mammography of a biopsy specimen (see Chapter 2).

In order to properly interpret either a mammogram or xeroradiogram a low-power magnifying lense is necessary for the detection of microcalcifications or fine stromal changes in the breast. Adequate interpretation of conventional mammograms requires a bright transilluminating light in addition to a magnifying lense. The skin line and adjacent subcutaneous tissues are examined with this technique. Xeroradiographs are read with reflected light and for optimal accuracy spectral characteristics similar to sunlight have been recommended. The examiner looks initially for the primary signs of malignancy—an irregular mass or microcalcifications. A benign tumor, such as a fibroadenoma, has relatively uniform density and well-defined margins which are often graphically demonstrated by a surrounding white halo due to edge enhancement on the xeroradiograph. There is usually no increase in vascularity around the benign lesion. Calcifications, if present in a benign lesion, are usually coarse and located around the periphery of the lesion. In contrast, malignant tumors have a poorly defined border, with spiculated or irregular areas usually without a white halo on the xeroradiograph (Fig. 3-1). Fine-stippled microcalcifications may be scattered throughout the tumor (Fig. 3-2). The venous pattern around a malignant tumor may also be increased. In some cases no mass may be apparent and the fine-stippled calcifications may be the only manifestation of a malignant tumor (Figs. 3-3 & 3-4). A unilateral prominent ductal pattern (asymmetrical ductal collagenosis) may be an early finding in neoplasia, and an extensive search of the radiograph for an underlying tumor must be undertaken. Secondary signs of malignancy include thickening of the overlying skin, skin retraction, nipple retraction, and obliteration of the retromammary space. These changes are usually only present in clinically obvious breast cancers.

If a lesion detected by mammography or xeroradiography is not palpable, it must be localized prior to surgical excision. Since cephalo-caudad and lateral views are routinely taken, it is generally possible to localize the lesion in respect to both the nipple and the margin of the breast. The location of the lesion is then indicated in relation to the face of a clock, i.e., at 10 o'clock 4 cm from the nipple and 3 cm deep to the skin.

Once the specimen is removed, the surgeon and pathologist must be sure that the radiographic abnormality has been included in the biopsy specimen (1, 3). The presence of the radiographic lesion in the specimen can be confirmed by a variety of techniques (14). One method is to inject contrast material, such as lipoidal, into the breast

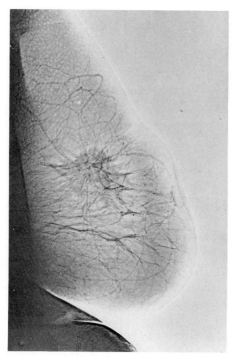 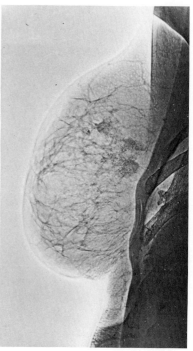

Fig. 3-1. Xeroradiogram (*lateral view*). The film demonstrates a spiculated mass with an irregular border and skin retraction superior to the nipple. Diagnosis—Scirrhous duct carcinoma.

Fig. 3-2. Xeroradiogram (*lateral view*). The film demonstrates multiple stippled calcifications. Some of the calcifications are within the mass, some are scattered around the mass. Diagnosis—Carcinoma.

tissue surrounding the radiographic lesion prior to biopsy. A radiography of the biopsy specimen is then made and the presence of contrast material in the tissue confirms the correct location of the biopsy. Another method of localization of the radiographic lesion is by placement of a fine needle under local anesthesia prior to the biopsy procedure (Fig. 3-5A,B,C). Methylene blue or some other indicator dye is then injected down along the needle tract. A third method of localization is to produce a radiograph of the biopsy specimen to compare with preoperative mammographic studies. Small masses or microcalcifications may be difficult however to detect with routine specimen mammography. As indicated in Chapter 2, our experience indicates that a xeroradiogram of the operative specimen constructs the optimal comparative image and vividly

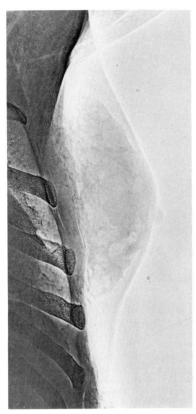
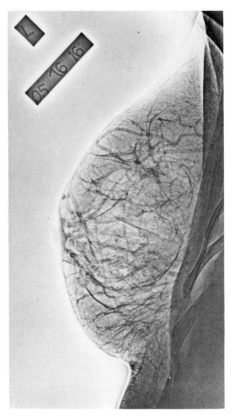

Fig. 3–3. Xeroradiogram. The film demonstrates multiple microcalcifitions in the inferior portion of the the breast carcinoma.

Fig. 3-4. Xeroradiogram. The film demonstrates multiple stippled calcifications in the inferior portion of the breast, no mass is present, the calcifications are the only sign of malignancy.

depicts very small tumor calcifications (Fig. 3–6A,B,C). The xeroradiographic process is no more time consuming than conventional radiography; any delay is thus usually determined by the proximity of the xeroradiographic unit to the operating room.

The indications for mammography or xeroradiography remain controversial. Wanebo (15) has demonstrated that irradiation can induce breast cancer and this danger of inducing malignant tumors limits the widespread use of these procedures.

Since the early 1960s technological innovations have been directed toward obtaining the desired diagnostic information in mam-

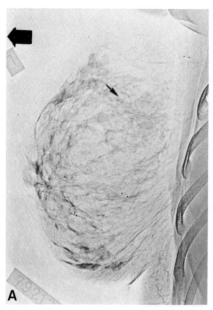

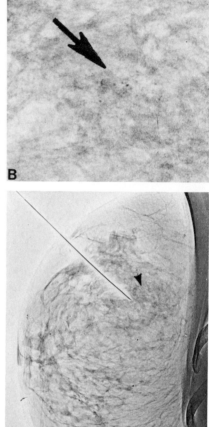

Fig. 3-5 A. Xeroradiogram (*lateral view*). The film demonstrates fibrocystic disease with a small area of microcalcifications (*arrow*) which are suspicious for an early carcinoma. No other signs of malignancy are seen. **B.** Xeroradiogram. Same patient with close-up view of the microcalcifications. **C.** Xeroradiogram (*lateral view*). The same patient with introduction of a 22 G localizing needle and injection of methylene blue.

mography with a minimum of radiation exposure to the patient. These include introduction of molybdenum targets, molybdenum filters, and beryllium windows for X-ray tubes, small focal spot tubes, and special image receptors (low-dose film mammography and xeroradiography). In our opinion xeromammography is the procedure of choice because of the considerable image content obtained by this technique and the relatively low-dose irradiation. A

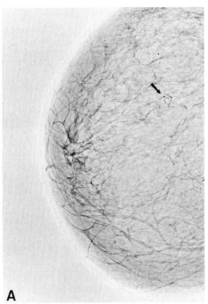

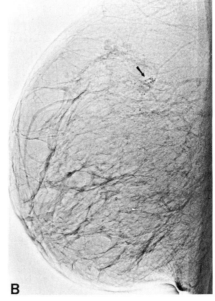

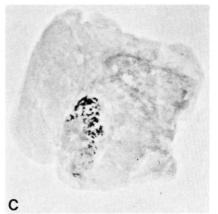

Fig. 3-6. **A, B.** Xeroradiogram (*ceph-alo-caudad and lateral view*) with a suspicious cluster of microcalcifications, depicted as dark specks. **C.** Specimen xeroradiogram. The cluster of microcalcifications are easily seen in this close-up view of the biopsy specimen from the patient in sections **A** and **B**.

method of automatic exposure termination has also been devised for xeromammography, which reduces the number of repeat exposures due to miscalculation of the proper exposure factors utilizing manual techniques (11). Either low-dose mammography or xeromammography should not be performed without specific indications in women under fifty years of age. Those women with a significant risk of developing breast cancer should probably be screened at two-to three-year intervals beginning at age thirty-five, particularly if they have large breasts with extensive fatty infiltration in which clinical detection of small masses by palpation is very difficult. This high-risk group of patients includes women with a positive family history of breast cancer and women who have never been pregnant. Those women with histologic evidence of a premalignant lesion on a previous breast biopsy also fall into this high-risk group of patients. All women over fifty should be screened at yearly intervals. Xeromammography should be considered in certain other carefully selected patients. The patient with severe symptomatic fibrocystic disease, manifested by pain and tenderness in association with an indiscrete mass, falls into this group. Xeromammography is performed as an aid in determining whether these lesions should be biopsied and also in which area to biopsy. Patients with known breast cancer who are candidates for a partial mastectomy are also screened by xeromammography in an effort to rule out other areas of occult cancer in the same breast. Xeromammography may also be utilized in the preoperative evaluation of patients with a mass clinically suggestive of cancer, in order to exclude a second clinically occult neoplastic site either within the breast containing the palpable mass or in the opposite breast.

Thermography

In 1956 Lawson (6) made the observation that breast cancers were associated with elevation of temperature in the skin overlying the cancer. This observation led to the development of photographic equipment which transferred the infra-red heat pattern of the skin of the breast to a visual display which can be photographed, thus producing a permanent record of the heat pattern of that particular breast. These films are then interpreted by comparing various shades of gray.

Thermography will detect certain breast cancers if the thermal gradient between the tumor and surrounding breast tissue is of sufficient magnitude to be detected by the infra-red photography. It should be noted, of course, that a thermogram only records the presence of increased heat. Localized areas of increased temperature are not pathognomonic of a malignant tumor; they may be due to a variety of other causes including an inflammatory reaction or increased venous blood flow.

If thermography proves to be an effective method of screening patients for breast cancer (8), it has the distinct advantage of avoiding irradiation and thus can be employed at frequent intervals in any type of patient. At the present time, however, there are several features of the technique which limit its usefulness. Temperature asymmetry is nonspecific. Some small tumors may not cause an increase in skin temperature overlying them. The interpretation of the photographs requires some experience in this technique and the incidence of false-positive readings remains rather high even in experienced hands. In order to obtain accurate photographs, the patient must be placed in a draft-free temperature-controlled environment, a requirement which is time-consuming and also necessitates a specially constructed room.

The concept of thermography is intriguing, and further investigations currently in progress may produce more meaningful data regarding its usefulness. At the present time, thermography is not considered to be a reliable technique for detecting breast cancer.

Mammary Duct Injections

This radiographic procedure is not employed as a screening technique. It is only performed in patients with a serous or bloody discharge from the nipple as a means of localizing its source (10).

The procedure is performed by squeezing the nipple and body of the breast to elicit a discharge in order to identify the ductal orifice. A small cannula is then introduced into the duct through which one-half to two mls of water-soluble contrast material is injected until the patient feels a pressure sensation. A radiograph of the breast in two projections is then performed immediately. An intraductal papilloma or an intraductal carcinoma can produce a filling defect in the involved duct and thus localize the source of the nipple discharge. This procedure is only indicated if the source of the nipple discharge cannot be localized to a specific quadrant of the breast by physical examination (Chapter 4).

References

1. Bauermeister, D. E., and Hall, M. H. 1973. Specimen radiography—a mandatory adjuvant to mammography. *Am. J. Clin. Pathol.* 59:782.
2. Boag, J. W. 1973. Xeroradiography. *Phys. Med. Biol.* 18:3–37.
3. Egan, R. L. 1964. *Mammography.* Springfield, Ill.: C. C. Thomas.
4. Gershon-Cohen, J., Hermel, M. B., and Birsner, J. W. 1970. Advances in mammographic technique. *Am. J. Roentgen.* 108:424.
5. Gilbertson, J. D., Randall, M. G., and Fingerhut, A. G. 1970. Evaluation of roentgen exposure in mammography. Part I. *Radiology* 95:383. Part II. *Radiology* 97:641.

6. Lawson, R. N. 1956. Implications of surface temperatures in the diagnosis of breast cancer. *Canad. Med. Ass. J.* 75:309.
7. LeBorgne, R. 1951. Diagnosis of tumors of the breast by simple roentgenography: Calcifications in carcinoma. *Am. J. Roentgen.* 65:1.
8. Lilienfeld, A. M., Barnes, J. M., Narnes, R. B., Brasfield, R., Connel, J. F., Diamond, E., Gershon-Cohen, J., Haberman, J., Isard, H. J., Lane, W. Z., Latter, R., Miller, J., Seaman, W., and Sherman, R. 1969. An evaluation of thermography in the detection of breast cancer. Cancer 24:1206.
9. Martin, J. E. 1973. Xeroradiography—an improved diagnostic method. *Am. J. Roentgen.* 117:1, 90–96.
10. Nunnerley, H. B., and Field, S. 1972. Mammary duct injection in patients with nipple discharge. *Brit. J. Radiology* 45:717.
11. Osterman, F. A., Zeman, G., Rao, G., and James, A. 1975. Xeroradiographic automatic exposure termination. *Radiology* (submitted). RSNA presentation, 1975.
12. Ostrum, B. J., Becker, W., Isard, H. J. 1973. Low dose mammography. *Radiology* 109:323.
13. Strax, P., Venet, L., and Shapiro, S. 1973. Value of mammography and reduction of mortality from breast cancer and mass screnning. *Amer. J. Roentgen., Radium Ther. Nuclear Med.* 117:3.
14. Synder, R. G., and Rosen, P. 1971. Radiology of breast specimens. *Cancer* 28:1608.
15. Wanebo, C. K., Johnson, K. G., and Sato, K., et al. 1968. Breast cancer after exposure to the atomic bombings of Hiroshima and Nagasaki. *New Engl. J. Med.* 279:667.

4. THE CLINICAL MANAGEMENT OF PRIMARY BREAST CANCER

R. Robinson Baker

Clinical Assessment

The initial clinical assessment of a patient with a breast mass is designed to determine the likelihood of malignancy. If the mass is thought to be malignant, the examiner also attempts to determine the growth rate of the tumor, the location and extent of the tumor within the breast, the presence or absence of regional lymph node metastases, the presence or absence of distant metastases, the virulence of the tumor, and evidence of host resistance. Since the presence of significant associated disease, such as congestive heart failure or chronic obstructive pulmonary disease, often significantly influences the type of therapy recommended for the breast cancer, the patient's general condition must also be assessed. The patient's response to the knowledge that she might have a breast cancer and her response to the possibility of losing her breast are also important components of the overall clinical assessment.

History. Malignant tumors probably do not increase in size at a constant rate and it is entirely possible that a small tumor may lie relatively dormant for a number of years prior to a rapid-growth phase. The rapid-growth phase may be due to some intrinsic property in the tumor, or it may be related to a change in host resistance, conceivably a breakdown in some type of immune surveillance system. In some cases, the growth rate of a malignant breast tumor can be relatively accurately determined by questioning the patient regarding the length of time the tumor has been present and how rapidly it has increased in size. The growth rate of the primary tumor may be of prognostic significance. For example, a 6-cm tumor which has been gradually increasing in size for several years, probably has a better prognosis than a 3-cm tumor which the patient is reasonably sure has doubled in size within the past month. The duration of symptoms is only one aspect of the history. Certain other specific inquiries should also be made relating to the menstrual history, family history, reproductive history, and past history of breast disease. All of this information is helpful in determining the possible etiology of the breast mass in question. A mass in the breast of a premenopausal woman is most likely a benign tumor or cyst. A mass in the breast of a postmenopausal woman is more likely to be a malignant tumor, particularly if the mass has recently appeared. The chances of the mass being a malignant tumor increase as the time interval from the menopause increases. A positive family history of breast cancer increases the chances that the mass is a malignant tumor. If the patient has never been pregnant the chances of breast cancer increase. The risk of breast cancer also increases as the age of the first pregnancy increases. In addition to the history relating to the duration of symptoms and various aspects of the menstrual and reproductive history, specific inquiries about possible symptoms of systemic metastases should also be made. The most common sites of systemic metastases are the mediastinal lymph nodes, lung parenchyma, pleura, spine, ribs, pelvis, and proximal femora. Pain from osseous metastases is the most common symptom of metastatic disease. Parenchymal lung metastases and pleural metastases can produce shortness of breath or vague chest pain. Mediastinal lymph node metastases can produce wheezing secondary to a partial obstruction of the trachea and/or dysphagia secondary to esophageal obstruction. Occasionally the first indication of a breast cancer is a pathologic fracture secondary to an osseous metastases.

Physical Examination. The physical examination is an important component of the clinical assessment, and a few words about how to perform the physical examination seem warranted. The physical examination should be accomplished in a systematic fashion with the patient in both the upright and the supine position, stripped to the waist in the presence of adequate light. Inspection prior to palpation is important, particularly with the patient in the upright position, first with her arms at her sides and then with her arms extended above her head. Inspection should also be performed while she is sitting slightly forward. Following initial inspection, the supraclavicular fossae are examined, with the head flexed to the ipsilateral side and then to the contralateral side. The axillae are examined with the pectoralis major muscle relaxed by adducting and supporting the arm. The nipple is examined for evidence of discharge, excoriation or ulceration. The breast is carefully palpated in a radial fashion with the tips of the fingers. The patient is asked to lie down and the breast is again carefully inspected. A careful radial examination is performed by light palpation. Deeper, more vigorous palpation is then performed to try to elicit a discharge from the nipple.

The majority of breast cancers are detected by the patient, who discovers an asymptomatic mass in her breast. Discrete mobile masses which are circumscribed and distinct from the adjacent breast tissue, particularly in the premenopausal woman, are more likely a fibroadenoma or a cyst. Malignant tumors are usually less distinct, and a three-dimensional impression is more difficult to obtain with a malignant tumor because of infiltration into the surrounding breast tissue. The degree of induration is not particularly helpful in differentiating benign from malignant tumors. Extreme induration usually indicates underlying malignancy, but extreme induration can also be present in a partially calcified fibroadenoma. The examining physician should measure the size of the mass and localize it to a specific quadrant of the breast. The proximity of the mass to the nipple is also determined. The majority of breast cancers are located in the upper outer quadrant or beneath the nipple. The increased incidence of malignant tumors in these areas is probably due to the fact that the majority of breast tissue is usually found there, i.e., more tissue is at risk in these locations. Cystic disease is also more commonly encountered in the upper outer quadrant of the breast and beneath the nipple.

Once the presence of a mass has been confirmed, measured, and located in a specific quadrant of the breast, other physical findings should be specifically looked for to continue the process of clinical assessment. These findings are almost always associated with a malignant tumor and indicate the presence of a locally invasive cancer. Skin retraction is due to involvement of the suspensory ligaments of the breast by infiltrating tumor. Fixation of the tumor to the pectoral musculature or to the chest wall also indicate the presence of an extensive infiltrating tumor which has invaded these adjacent structures. The examiner also looks for other changes in the skin of the breast, particularly dimpling of the skin, erythema of the overlying skin, or the presence of satellite nodules in the skin of the breast several centimeters away from the palpable primary tumor.

Dimpling of the skin (peau d'orange change) indicates the presence of a tumor which has invaded the dermal lymphatics. Dermal lymphatic invasion is a sign of a very aggressive cancer which has almost always metastasized to distant organs.

A malignant tumor which produces erythema of the skin is by definition an inflammatory breast cancer. The term inflammatory breast cancer is a clinical rather than a pathologic description of the breast, and is a confusing and misleading term because of the wide variation in clinical signs which have been referred to as "inflammatory." Any tumor which is associated with warmth, tenderness, edema, erythema, or ulceration can be referred to as an inflammatory breast cancer, but all of these physical signs are not associated with the same prognosis. In the past, most authorities on breast cancer have considered inflammatory breast cancer to be incurable. Ellis and Teitelbaum (14) have recently pointed out, however, that all inflammatory breast cancers are not necessarily fatal. Only those tumors with dermal lymphatic metastases are universally fatal; other inflammatory breast cancers are not uniformly fatal and a five-year survival rate in the range of 10 to 15 percent has been reported with inflammatory breast cancers which do not involve the dermal lymphatics. The exact cause of erythema of the skin in association with a breast cancer is not known, but it is not due to bacterial infection. Grace and Dayo (22) have presented experimental work that indicates that the patient is allergic to the tumor and that the erythema is due to a hypersensitivity reaction. This theory is supported by a number of experiments in patients with inflammatory breast cancer who received intradermal injections of autologous tumor extracts. All of these patients developed an inflammatory reaction in the skin overlying the autologous tumor implant. In contrast, none of the control patients with noninflammatory breast cancer who received intradermal injections of autologous tumor extracts developed an inflammatory reaction in the overlying skin.

The presence of satellite skin nodules indicates that cells from the primary breast cancer have invaded blood vessels and/or lymphatics and emboli of tumor cells have implanted in the adjacent skin. Past experience has indicated that these findings are almost invariably associated with other foci of distant metastases and therefore these patients are incurable.

Excoriation of the nipple may indicate Paget's disease of the nipple, which is invariably associated with an underlying intraductal carcinoma and sometimes with infiltrating carcinoma as well. The intraductal carcinoma may or may not be palpable and the excoriated nipple may be the only indication of its presence. A specific diagnosis of Paget's disease can be confirmed by a small incisional biopsy of the nipple. A discharge from the nipple is usually not an indication of malignancy in the premenopausal woman. Serous or mucus discharges can be smeared for cytologic study and, if the smear is negative for malignant cells, no therapy is necessary. Since serous or mucus discharges from the nipple are rarely caused by malignancy, a cytologic diagnosis of malignancy should be confirmed by excision of the quadrant of the breast which was the source of the nipple discharge and the cytologic diagnosis confirmed by histologic examination. If a bloody discharge from the nipple is detected, careful radial palpation is performed. The location of the underlying lesions can usually be detected in this fashion, i.e., palpation of one specific area causes the bloody discharge from the nipple. This area is excised for histologic study and the histologic sections usually confirm the presence of an intraductal papilloma. If the source of the bloody discharge is not located by radial palpation, a xeroradiogram is obtained in an effort to detect a mass. In the absence of xeroradiographic evidence of a mass, radio-opaque dye is injected into the ductal system and X-rays obtained in an effort to localize the source of bleeding. If a lesion is detected it can be excised. If no lesion is detected and the cytologic smear reveals no evidence of malignancy the patient is asked to return for physical examination at three-month intervals. The radiographic procedures are repeated at yearly intervals. A serous or bloody discharge from the nipple of a postmenopausal woman is more suspicious of malignancy, although an intraductal papilloma may also be encountered in a postmenopausal woman. Similar diagnostic procedures are performed to localize the source of the serous or bloody discharge. If all of these studies reveal no evidence of malignancy, frequent follow-up examinations are indicated until the source of the bleeding or discharge is localized.

Palpable axillary lymph nodes do not necessarily contain metastatic cancer. The examiner must make a judgment on the basis of the clinical findings whether he thinks the axillary lymph nodes contain metastatic tumor. Small, soft, slightly tender nodes usually do not contain metastatic tumor. Indurated, rubbery nodes usually do contain metastatic tumor. Fixation of the nodes to each other or to the skin overlying the axilla is almost invariably due to metastatic cancer within the node. The nodes become fixed because the tumor has grown through the capsule of the node and invaded adjacent structures. Metastatic tumors growing out of the axillary nodes can also obstruct vessels draining the arm and eventually the axillary or subclavian vein. Edema of the arm is thus another physical sign of advanced breast cancer.

The supraclavicular fossae should be carefully palpated. Palpable lymph nodes greater than 1.5 cms in diameter usually contain metastatic tumor, but the examiner should remember that the lung or gastrointestinal tract may be the source of the primary tumor. Visible or palpable internal mammary lymph nodes are unusual, except in advanced cases of breast cancer.

Further clinical assessment is dependent upon the findings on the history and physical examination. If the patient is premenopausal, and a clinical diagnosis of either a fibroadenoma or cyst has been established, additional radiographic studies are not indicated, and the next maneuver is designed to establish a definitive histologic diagnosis. In a woman under age thirty a nontender, freely mobile mass is usually a fibroadenoma. Excisional biopsy under local anesthesia is performed to remove the mass and establish a histologic diagnosis. If the mass fluctuates in size and is associated with slight pain and tenderness, the diagnosis of a cyst can be confirmed by needle aspiration. The fluid obtained by aspiration is sent to a cytology laboratory to rule out the presence of malignant cells. The patient is examined six weeks later to determine whether the cyst has refilled. If the cyst has recurred, it is excised. If needle aspiration fails to obtain fluid, excisional biopsy under local anesthesia is indicated to establish a histologic diagnosis.

Radiographic Studies

Xeroradiograms and mammograms are primarily screening procedures and should not be employed as diagnostic procedures in the management of patients with a palpable breast mass. A palpable mass should be either aspirated for cytologic study or excised for histologic study, regardless of what it appears to be on xeroradiography or mammography. Although these X-ray procedures can detect both clinically palpable and clinically occult malignant tumors, a few breast cancers cannot be demonstrated by either xeroradiography or mammography, and the patient and her physician should not be lulled into a false sense of security if the palpable mass is either not visualized or does not appear to have the radiographic characteristics of malignancy. Although xeroradiograms and/or mammograms should not be obtained as an aid in the diagnosis of a palpable mass, I see no objection to obtaining these studies in patients over forty-five years of age who are undergoing a breast biopsy. These preoperative or prebiopsy radiographic studies are obtained to detect the presence of clinically occult lesions in either breast, so that they can be biopsied when the palpable mass is excised. If the palpable mass proves to be a carcinoma, the xeroradiogram or mammogram of the opposite breast can be compared to any subsequent radiographic procedures obtained during the follow-up period.

In any patient with a mass which is clinically suspicious of malignancy or a biopsy-proven breast cancer, a chest X-ray is obtained prior to definitive treatment in order to detect asymptomatic metastatic lesions in the lung parenchyma, pleura, or skeletal structures visualized. The chest X-ray is not a particularly sensitive method of detecting metastatic disease, since pulmonary parenchymal lesions must be at least 1 cm to 2 cms in size before they are demonstrable on the chest X-ray, and metastatic bone lesions are not demonstrable until 50 to 75 percent of the mineral content of the bone has been lost.

The skeletal system, a common site for metastatic breast cancer, is also surveyed for occult metastases. Three methods of screening the skeletal system are available, the serum alkaline phosphatase, X-rays of bones most likely to contain metastatic lesions, and bone scans.

An elevated serum alkaline phosphatase in the presence of other normal liver chemistries usually indicates either bone metastases or liver metastases. The presence of metastatic disease in the liver may be detected by a liver scan or needle biopsy. The detection of bone metastases is discussed in the next paragraph.

A bone survey consists of X-rays of bones which are most likely to be invaded by metastatic breast cancer. These bones are in order of decreasing frequency, the ribs, sternum, lumbar spine, skull, proximal femora, and thoracic spine. A bone survey is not a sensitive technique for detecting early bone metastases because as previously noted, 50 to 75 percent of the mineral content of the bone must be lost before the metastatic focus becomes roentgenographically apparent as a radiolucency. Several investigators (4, 27) have demonstrated that at least 50 percent of the skeletal metastases from breast cancer found at autopsy were not apparent on X-rays taken shortly before the patient died. For these reasons, I believe that screening for occult bone metastases by X-ray alone is a useless procedure.

Bone scans, particularly when employed in conjunction with X-rays, are a more sensitive means of detecting small bone metastases. A bone scan is obtained with a rectilinear scanner or Anger gamma camera after the intravenous injection of isotopes which localize in bones. Technetium 99m labeled polyphosphate and diphosphate, which has a half-life of six hours and delivers only minimal irradiation to the bone, is the most commonly employed radiopharmaceutical at the present time. An increased concentration of isotope will occur in any area of new bone formation and also in any area where the regional perfusion is increased. Increased concentration of isotope is not therefore pathognomonic of metastatic bone disease and the bone scan must be interpreted in conjunction with X-rays and associated clinical findings. Roentgenograms are frequently of use in determining the etiology of the abnormal isotope concentration. In 70 to 80 percent of the patients with breast cancer and an abnormal bone scan, roentgenograms, either plain X-rays and/or tomograms, will confirm the presence of a metastatic lesion or demonstrate some other abnormality, such as osteoarthritis, which would explain the increased concentration of isotope. The patient with an abnormal bone scan and no X-ray evidence of a bony lesion is more difficult to evaluate. This situation occurs in 15 to 20 percent of patients with breast cancer and an abnormal bone scan. If the tomograms are also normal a judgment must be made as to the possible etiology of the area of new bone formation or increased regional perfusion. A history of arthritis or trauma to the area indicates a possible benign lesion which would have a small focus of new bone formation. Multiple myeloma or some other type of primary or metastatic malignant lesion should also be considered. If there is no other clinical or radiographic evidence of another lesion, the lesion in question is probably an occult metastatic breast tumor. In a very small number of patients, X-rays will reveal an abnormality which is normal on bone scintigraphy. This situation occurs most often in the presence of osteoblastic metastatic breast lesions.

The indications for preoperative bone scans in patients with clinically suspicious or biopsy proven breast cancer have not been precisely defined. Galasko (21) reports an abnormal bone scan in 24 percent of fifty patients with operable breast cancer, but the clinical stage of disease of these patients is not defined. El-Domeiri (13) divides a group of fifty-five patients into various clinical stages of disease and correlates the clinical stage with the incidence of an abnormal bone scan. Only one out of twenty-four patients with T_1 and T_2 lesions (see section on Clinical Staging, p. 85-87) had an abnormal bone scan. In contrast, 40 percent of patients with T_3 lesions had abnormal bone scans. In our experience, an occasional patient with a T_1 or T_2 lesion without evidence of axillary lymph node metastases has had an abnormal bone scan which on further X-ray examination appears to be due to metastatic breast cancer (Fig. 4-1). The incidence of positive bone scans in patients with Stages I and II breast cancer, however, is low, probably 5 percent. Preoperative bone scans are not recommended routinely, therefore, in all patients with Stages I and II disease. They should be performed in all patients with Stage III disease, because the incidence of occult bone metastases in this group of patients is considerably higher.

Laboratory Findings. A routine preoperative workup includes a hematocrit and white blood cell count. Both of these studies are usually within normal limits. Metastatic disease may produce anemia secondary to bone marrow replacement or suppression, but this type of anemia is almost always associated with extensive clinical evidence of metastatic disease. Since the liver and bones are common sites of metastatic tumor, a serum alkaline phosphatase is obtained as a screening procedure for metastatic bone or liver disease as previously noted.

Clinical Staging. When the clinical assessment has been completed, the clinical stage of the disease can be determined. Clinical staging has been developed to provide guide lines as to therapy and also a means of comparing two different methods of therapy in a group of patients with the same stage of disease. The following method of clinical staging has been slightly modified from the clinical staging proposed by the National Surgical Adjuvant Breast Project. In this clinical staging the letter "T" refers to the primary tumor, the letter "N" refers to the regional lymph nodes, and the letter "M" refers to distant metastases. The methods of clinical staging and the clinical stages are outlined below.

"T" Primary Tumor

T0 No palpable lesion (includes those lesions detected by mammography and xeroradiography).

T1 Tumor 2 cms or less in greatest dimension.
 Skin not involved, except in the case of Paget's disease confined to nipple.
 No retraction of nipple.
 No pectoral muscle fixation.
 No chest wall attachment.

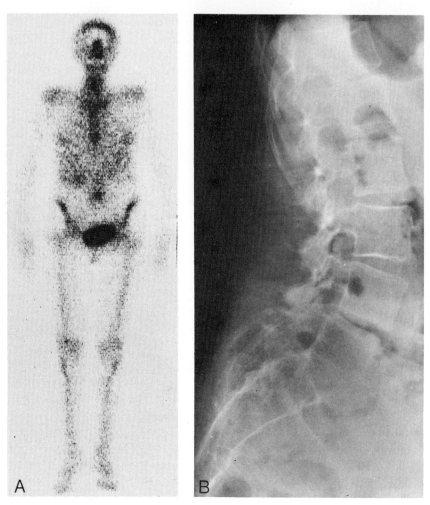

Fig. 4–1. **A.** Bone scan demonstrating increased activity in the lumbar spine. The patient had a 2-cm asymptomatic carcinoma of the left breast and a clinically negative left axilla. **B.** X-ray of the lumbar spine of the same patient. The X-ray demonstrates a large lytic lesion in the 3rd lumbar vertebra.

T2   Tumor over 2 cms in greatest dimension without skin involvement.
       Tumor of any size with any of the following signs of skin involvement:
             incomplete skin fixation (tethering or dimpling, i.e., movable over the tumor).

nipple retraction (subaureolar tumor), or

Paget's disease extending beyond the nipple, or

ulceration of less than 2 cms in its greatest dimension if there is no histologic evidence of dermal lymphatic invasion.

No pectoral muscle fixation.

No chest wall attachment.

T3 Tumor of any size with any of the following:

complete fixation of skin to underlying tumor, i.e., skin not movable;

ulceration greater than 2 cms in its greatest dimensions, but not associated with histologic evidence of dermal lymphatic invasion.

Pectoral muscle fixation (complete or incomplete).

Chest wall attachment.

"N" Regional Lymph Nodes

N0 No clinically palpable axillary lymph nodes.

N1 Clinically palpable axillary lymph nodes 2 cms or less in greatest dimension.

1a. Palpable nodes not considered to contain tumor (metastases not suspected) that are moveable in relation to the chest wall and other structures.

1b. Palpable nodes considered to contain tumor (metastases suspected) that are moveable or fixed to one another, but not greater than 2 cms and not fixed to any other structures.

N2 Axillary lymph nodes in excess of 2 cms in greatest dimension.

Axillary lymph nodes fixed to other structures.

N3 Supra- or infraclavicular nodes, moveable or fixed.

Edema of the arm.

"M" Distant Metastases

M0 No distant metastases.

M1 Distant Metastases present (clinical or radiographic evidence).

1a. Skin involvement wide of breast, including clinical evidence or peau d'orange change or erythema or ulceration of the breast, which is associated with histologic evidence of dermal lymphatic invasion.

    1b. Involvement of contralateral nodes or contralateral breast.

    1c. Clinical or radiographic evidence of metastases to lungs, pleural cavity, skeleton, liver, etc.

Clinical Stages

Stage I	Stage II	Stage III	Stage IV
T0 N0 M0	T0 N1b M0	T0 N2 M0	Any combination
T1 N0 M0	T1 N1b M0	T1 N2 M0	of T and N with
T2 N0 M0	T2 N1b M0	T2 N2 M0	M1
T0 N1a M0		T3 N0 M0	
T1 N1a M0		T3 N1a M0	
T2 N1a M0		T3 N1b M0	
		T3 N2 M0	
		T1 N3 M0	
		T2 N3 M0	
		T3 N3 M0	

The ten-year survival rates according to the various stages of disease are reviewed in Fig. 4–2. The ten-year survival rate of patients with Stage I disease is approximately 80 percent. The ten-year survival rate of patients with Stage II disease is in the range of 50 percent. Thirty percent of those patients with Stage III disease will survive for ten years. The great majority of patients with Stage IV disease are dead within five years, all of these patients are dead within ten years. This method of clinical staging includes one group of patients who, in the past, have been classified as Stage IV disease. These are patients with supraclavicular or infraclavicular lymph node metastases (N3). Although a few of these patients will survive for long periods of time after irradiation, the percentage is very small.

In spite of this very detailed system of clinical staging, wide variations in survival rates occur within each clinical stage. This variation occurs for a number of reasons. There is a 30 percent chance of error in placing the patients in Clinical Stage I versus Clinical Stage II, i.e., 30 percent of the patients with clinically negative nodes will have histologically positive nodes, and an equal number of patients with clinically positive nodes will have histologically negative nodes. Patients with no evidence of metastatic disease are placed in Stage II. As previously noted, X-rays and other methods of screening patients for possible metastatic disease are relatively insensitive in detecting small metastases. As a result, a

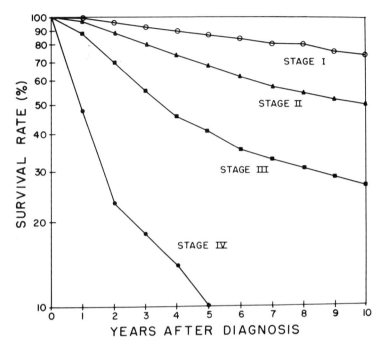

Fig. 4-2. Percentage of patients surviving at yearly intervals correlated with stage of disease.

large number of patients who are classified as having Stage II disease really have Stage IV disease, but these occult metastases cannot be found by presently available screening techniques. Wide variations in survival rates within the same clinical stage of disease are also due to variations in the virulence of the tumor and in host resistance. Current methods of clinical staging do not consider either of these factors.

Histology. An estimate of the virulence of the primary tumor can be made after a histologic examination of the biopsy specimen. As noted in Chapter 2, certain histologic patterns, such as medullary carcinoma, colloid carcinoma, papillary carcinoma, comedocarcinoma and tubular carcinoma, are associated with considerably better survival rates than the survival rates obtained after treatment of the more common scirrhous duct carcinomas. In addition to the histologic patterns, other histologic criteria give some indication of the virulence of a particular tumor (Chapter 2). On the basis of histologic features, such as nuclear configuration, the number of mitoses and the size of the nucleoli, each tumor may be assigned a histologic grade. Tumors containing cells with large pleomorphic nuclei, large nucleoli, prominent nuclear membranes, and numerous mitoses are classified as high-grade tumors. This type of tumor is associated with relatively low survival rates, regardless of clinical stage. In contrast, tumors with small nuclei, barely visible nucleoli, and few mitoses are classified as low-grade tumors. This type of tumor is associated with considerably better survival rates, again regardless of clinical stage.

There are other histologic findings which may provide some insight into the interaction between the tumor and the host. Histologic evidence of round cell infiltration around the primary tumor and the histologic appearance of the axillary lymph nodes which do not contain metastases may give some indication of host resistance, but, of course, these findings cannot be evaluated prior to treatment. The growth pattern of the tumor also appears to be of some significance; tumors with a circumscribed border which appears to be pushing the normal tissue ahead of the margin of the tumor have a better prognosis than tumors with an infiltrating growth pattern, as do carcinomas with a significant noninvasive component. A tumor with a viable cohesive pattern has a better prognosis than a tumor with extensive areas of necrosis.

Biopsy. Histologic study of the tumor can, of course, only be accomplished after biopsy. The timing of the biopsy is controversial. In the past, the usual approach has been to discuss the possibility of a mastectomy with the patient prior to operation, perform the biopsy under general anesthesia and proceed with some type of mastectomy if a frozen section of the tumor reveals a malignancy. In my opinion, this approach should be abandoned in most instances. General anesthesia carries a slight but definite risk and is not necessary in a large number of patients. Premenopausal women with clinically benign disease, such as a fibroadenoma or a cyst which cannot be decompressed by aspiration, are advised to have an excisional biopsy under local anesthesia as an out-patient, thus avoiding the risk of general anesthesia and the expense of two to three days in the hospital.

A premenopausal or postmenopausal woman with a breast mass which is clinically suspicious of malignancy can be managed in a variety of ways. Biopsy under general anesthesia is indicated in women who prefer general anesthesia and who are willing to undergo a definitive procedure following the frozen section diagnosis of the tumor. However, some women with suspicious clinical findings are not willing to go to sleep not knowing whether the mass in their breast is benign or malignant and whether they will wake up with a small incision or an absent breast. Biopsy under local anesthesia is performed in this particular group of women and further discussions as to the possible means of therapy are conducted after a histologic assessment of the tumor has been completed. Biopsy under local anesthesia is also indicated in patients in whom a partial mastectomy or subcutaneous mastectomy is being considered, since histologic evaluation of the tumor is an important consideration.

I am not aware of any disadvantage in biopsying malignant tumors under local anesthesia as long as care is taken not to insert the needle administering the local anesthetic through the malignant tumor and into the underlying fascia or muscle. If the tumor is malignant the entire biopsy area, including the overlying skin, is subsequently excised so that local implantation of tumor cells could not be of any significance. The theoretical possibility of injecting malignant cells into the lymphatic channels or blood vessels does exist, but in my opinion is negligible.

The technique of biopsy is important. If the lesion is near the nipple, a circumaureolar incision is performed because it heals with an excellent cosmetic result. If the lesion is not adjacent to the aureola, circumferential incisions over the tumor mass are performed because these incisions heal with a considerably better cosmetic result than radial incisions extending from the nipple to the periphery. It is important to place these incisions so that they will not compromise any subsequent mastectomy skin flaps. Excisional biopsies are generally preferred, but if the tumor is in close approximation to the underlying pectoral fascia, an incisional biopsy is performed to avoid implantation of the tumor cells into the underlying pectoral fascia. An increasing number of suspicious lesions are being detected by mammography and xeroradiography. In some of these cases, the lesion is too small to be localized by physical examination. Various methods of localizing the lesion prior to biopsy are discussed in detail in Chapter 3. Biopsy of nonpalpable lesions detected by mammography or xeroradiography should only be performed in an institution where some type of specimen radiography equipment is available. As noted in Chapter 3, we feel that specimen xeroradiography is the optimal means of confirming the presence of a specimen similar to that which was detected by the preoperative xeroradiogram.

If, following an excisional biopsy, there is a suspicion of malignancy on gross examination, only a small piece of tissue is submitted for histologic section and confirmation of the malignancy by the pathologist. The remainder of the tumor is frozen and later assayed for the presence or absence of specific proteins which bind estrogen and/or progesterone (estrogen and progesterone receptors). Similar studies are also performed on residual tumor in the mastectomy specimen if an incisional biopsy has established the diagnosis of carcinoma. The presence or absence of estrogen and progesterone receptors in a breast cancer does not influence primary therapy at the present time, but these studies are extremely useful in the management of patients with metastatic breast cancer (see Chapter 5). Such studies should be carried out on all primary tumors, because if metastatic lesions are detected at some future date they may not be accessible to excision and, therefore, these determinations for the presence or absence of estrogen and progesterone receptors could not be performed.

Summary of Clinical Assessment. It is important to recognize that breast cancer is a spectrum of disease. The opposite ends of the spectrum can be identified without difficulty and the subsequent clinical course of these patients predicted with reasonable accuracy. The center of the spectrum is the gray area. In this area the prediction of the subsequent clinical course on the basis of the clinical assessment is more difficult.

Tumors at the more favorable end of the spectrum have the following characteristics. They have been present for six to twelve months without noticeable change in size; they are less than 2.5 cm in size; there is no fixation to the skin or to the pectoral muscles; there is no clinical evidence of axillary or internal mammary or supraclavicular lymphadenopathy; the chest X-ray is normal; histologic sections of the tumor reveal a favorable histologic pattern or a scirrhous duct carcinoma of low histologic grade with pushing borders and no evidence of necrosis within the tumor. These patients will do well and survive for long periods of time after many different types of therapy. Tumors at the opposite end of the spectrum have doubled in size within a month, are greater than 4 cm in size, have produced erythema or actual ulceration of the overlying skin, are fixed to the pectoral muscles, and are associated with large axillary lymph nodes which may be fixed to the overlying skin. Histologic sections of these tumors usually reveal a poorly differentiated scirrhous duct carcinoma of high histologic grade, with infiltrative borders and multiple foci of necrosis. Although there may be no clinical or radiographic evidence of distant metastases, the majority of these patients are incurable because occult metastases are present. An even more unfavorable case is the woman who presents with a history of rapid ulceration of the breast and back pain, who proves to have a scirrhous duct carcinoma of high histologic grade and radiographic evidence of osseous and visceral metastases.

The closer one comes to the center of the spectrum where the majority of cases of breast cancer are located, the more difficult the prediction of subsequent behavior. These are the patients with a two- to three-month history of a mass in the breast, which measures somewhere between 2.5 cm and 4 cm in size and is not fixed to the skin or pectoral musculature. Axillary nodes may or may not be palpable, and the biopsy reveals a scirrhous duct carcinoma of intermediate histologic grade. The chest X-ray and bone scan reveal no evidence of metastases. Sixty to 70 percent of the patients with primary breast cancer will fall into this category. The subsequent clinical course is variable; if no axillary nodes contain metastatic breast carcinoma, approximately 75 percent of these patients will survive ten years. If axillary nodes are involved, the ten-year survival rate is approximately 30 percent.

Treatment

History. The surgical treatment of breast cancer prior to the latter half of the nineteenth century consisted primarily of local excision of the tumor. Surgeons usually encountered patients with large indolent tumors which had frequently ulcerated the overlying skin and had metastasized to the lymph nodes of the axilla. Local excision of these tumors was associated with a 50 to 80 percent incidence of local recurrence, and these results indicated that a more extensive procedure was necessary. Such a procedure was performed by Dr. William S. Halsted in 1882 (24). This operation, the radical mastectomy, was designed to excise the entire breast, the skin overlying the breast, the muscles underlying the breast, and to combine this excision with an en block or incontinuity dissection of the contents of the axilla. The original operation also excised the clavicle and supraclavicular lymph nodes, but he subsequently abandoned this extension of the procedure. The axillary lymph node dissection in association with the mastectomy had been performed earlier by Banks in England and Kuster in Germany, but Halsted certainly popularized the operation, particularly when he was able to reduce the recurrence rate in the scar of the operative procedure to

6 percent and the late regional recurrence rate to 16 percent. The radical mastectomy as described by Halsted was and continues to be an effective means of removing large indolent tumors confined to the chest wall and axilla. One should remember, however, that Halsted's knowledge of breast cancer and its mode of spread was considerably different from what is known about the disease in 1976. The patients who came to his attention had large indolent tumors which remained confined to the chest wall and axilla for prolonged periods of time. Forty-eight of his original fifty cases had axillary lymph node metastases. He was not aware that blood-borne metastases occurred and based his operation conceptually on the idea that breast cancer only metastasized via the lymphatics. Patients with small primary breast cancers and widespread metastatic disease secondary to blood-borne metastases probably never came to his attention.

After ninety years of intensive investigation, it is now apparent that breast cancer is a considerably different disease than was apparent in 1882, and that concepts concerning treatment should be modified accordingly. Breast cancer is conceivably due to a variety of etiologic agents. It certainly presents with a variety of histologic patterns, and it varies dramatically in its clinical course. There is no reason, therefore, to continue to routinely apply an operative procedure designed to eliminate one type of breast cancer to all types of breast cancer. If a particular case presents with a large indolent tumor confined to the chest wall and axilla, the radical mastectomy is an effective means of treating this particular type of tumor. The radical mastectomy should not, however, be routinely employed in the management of a small tumor of the breast without evidence of axillary metastases.

Within the past fifty years a number of different methods of therapy have been suggested, and numerous clinical trials have been reported. Some investigators have described less extensive surgical procedures in comparison to the radical mastectomy, either alone or in combination with irradiation. Other investigators have employed the radical mastectomy in only the most favorable cases, treating all other cases with irradiation. Another group of investigators have advocated extension of the operative procedures to include the internal mammary and supraclavicular nodes as well as the axillary nodes. Pre- and postoperative irradiation has been employed as an adjuvant to the radical mastectomy or extended radical mastectomy. As the result of these clinical trials, certain facts are evident. All patients dying of breast cancer, approximately 30,000 women in the United States in 1974, are dying of distant metastases. These metastases occur because the cells from certain malignant tumors are capable of invading blood vessels, gaining entrance into the systemic circulation, surviving within the systemic circulation and lodging at distant sites. A few of these circulating cells may gain entrance to the systemic circulation as a result of operative manipulation of the tumor, but the vast majority are either in the systemic circulation, or have become established as microscopic foci of metastases in the bone or other viscera, prior to treatment. More extensive local ablative procedures, i.e., larger operations or larger doses of irradiation alone or in combination with surgery will not, therefore, significantly increase survival rates. Survival rates will only increase if the breast cancers are detected prior to the occurrence of distant metastases or when effective methods of chemotherapy or immunotherapy are developed to destroy occult metastases.

Description of Various Methods of Therapy. Prior to any further discussion about the optimal means of treatment, various methods of therapy are briefly described to give the reader some indication of the morbidity and cosmetic deformities produced by these procedures.

The most conservative procedure is local excision of the tumor with a margin of normal breast tissue and an ellipse of skin overlying the tumor mass. This procedure has a variety of names; it is referred to as quadrant excision, lumpectomy, tylectomy, or partial mastectomy. The procedure should remove the primary tumor with a wide margin of normal breast tissue, the skin overlying the tumor, and pectoral fascia beneath the tumor. A variety of incisions can be employed, radial incisions for lesions in the outer quadrants and lesions medial to the nipple, transverse incisions for lesions above or below the nipple (Fig. 4-3). In women with relatively small breasts, the procedure can be performed under local anesthesia with little blood loss. Large breasts usually require a general anesthesia. Partial mastectomies produce varying deformities of the breast, depending upon the size of the breast and size and location of the tumor. The multifocal origin of breast cancer is the primary objection to this type of procedure. Shah, Gallagher, and Rosen (20, 39, 41) have demonstrated that breast cancer is a disease of multifocal origin, and therefore a quadrant excision or partial mastectomy which may excise the palpable mass with a margin of normal breast tissue does not necessarily remove all of the other foci of microscopic cancer. In Rosen's study (39) the quadrant containing the palpable mass was initially excised and then a radical mastectomy was

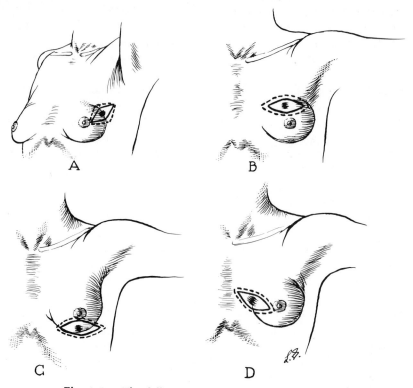

Fig. 4–3. The following incisions are recommended for a partial mastectomy. The *Solid line* indicates the extent of skin excision, the *dotted line* indicates the extent of excision of the breast tissue around the tumor mass. **A**—Lesion in the upper outer quadrant. **B**—Lesion above the nipple. **C**—Lesion below the nipple. **D**—Lesion in the inner quadrant.

performed and the remaining three quadrants of the breast submitted for histologic section. If the palpable lesion was less than 2 cm in size, 26 percent of the patients had carcinoma remaining in the residual breast after the simulated partial mastectomy. The incidence of residual carcinoma rose to 38 percent if the primary tumor was greater than 2 cm in size.

A somewhat more extensive procedure is a simple mastectomy, also referred to as a mastectomy or total mastectomy. This procedure removes the breast tissue including the nipple and skin overlying the tumor mass. In older women with pendulous breasts, a simple mastectomy can be easily accomplished under local anesthesia but this type of procedure usually does not remove all of the breast tissue. An absolute total mastectomy is a relatively time-consuming procedure which requires meticulous dissection of skin flaps in order to remove all the breast tissue from the overlying skin. In my experience a simple mastectomy usually does not remove all of the breast tissue unless the skin flaps are meticulously dissected or a skin graft is employed. The failure of most simple mastectomies to totally remove all of the breast tissue should be kept in mind when considering a subcutaneous mastectomy. The subcutaneous mastectomy also does not remove all of the breast tissue, but if carefully performed it probably removes as much breast tissue as the usual simple mastectomy.

A subcutaneous mastectomy excises the breast tissue but preserves the nipple and skin (Fig. 4-4). If carefully performed, 85 to 90 percent of the breast tissue can be excised. Residual foci of breast tissue are usually left beneath the nipple and along the superior and medial margins of the dissection. The subcutaneous mastectomy requires general anesthesia. The procedure is technically more difficult to perform than a partial mastectomy or a simple mastectomy and is associated with an appreciable blood loss. Following the subcutaneous mastectomy a Silastic implant can be inserted into the pocket left after excision of the breast tissue either simultaneously or at varying intervals following the subcutaneous mastectomy. A bilateral procedure is almost always necessary for a satisfactory cosmetic result. As previously noted a carefully performed subcutaneous mastectomy probably removes as much breast tissue as the usual simple mastectomy which does not employ a skin graft or the construction of extremely thin skin flaps. The subcutaneous mastectomy may devascularize the overlying skin, particularly in the lower outer quadrant of the breast. Approximately 10 percent of patients undergoing a carefully performed subcutaneous mastectomy will develop focal areas of skin necrosis if all of the breast tissue is excised from the overlying skin. The skin slough necessitates removal of the implant and excision of the necrotic skin. The Silastic implant can be reinserted four to six months later. Infection also occurs in a small percentage of patients, necessitating removal of the implants.

A mastectomy combined with an axillary node dissection but with preservation of the pectoral musculature is called a modified radical mastectomy (Fig. 4-5). This operation excises the nipple and skin overlying the tumor and all of the underlying breast tissue if thin skin flaps are employed. The fascia of the pectoralis major muscle is removed, the pectoralis minor muscle is divided, and an incontinuity

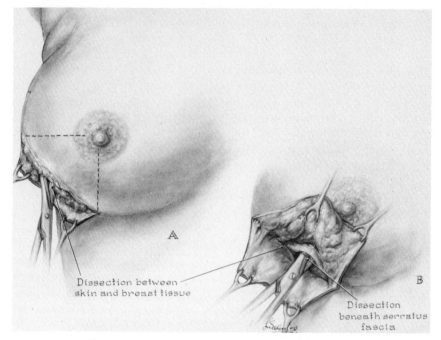

Dissection between
skin and breast tissue

A

B

Dissection
beneath serratus
fascia

Fig. 4-4. **A.** A circumferential incision is made in the inframammary fold of the lower outer quadrant of the breast. **B.** The dissection is carried down beneath the fascia of the anterior serratus muscle. **C.** The dissection is continued beneath the breast tissue, beginning a plane of dissection between the breast tissue and the fascia of the pectoralis major muscle. It is very important to develop this plane of dissection anterior to the fascia of the pectoralis major muscle. **D.** The entire breast is mobilized away from the fascia of the pectoralis major muscle by blunt, finger dissection. **E.** The dissection beneath the breast is continued up to the second rib superiorly and medially to the costal cartilages, utilizing long dissecting scissors as necessary. (Continued on next page)

axillary lymph node dissection is performed. The cosmetic defect produced is similar to that following a simple mastectomy without an axillary node dissection. If the procedure is performed through a transverse incision, the cosmetic and functional result is considerably better than that obtained following a radical mastectomy performed through a vertical incision. Later reconstruction with a Silastic implant is feasible. Swelling of the ipsilateral arm (lymphedema) occurs in approximately 10 percent of the cases and is due to damage to the lymphatic vessels draining the arm. The only other significant complication is related to healing of the skin flaps. If all of the breast tissue is removed from beneath the skin flaps, the skin

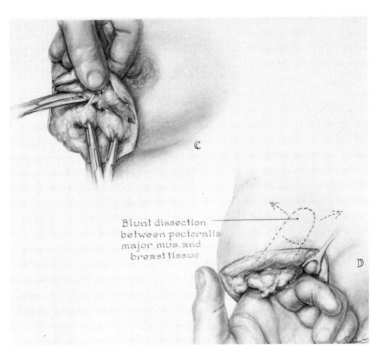

Blunt dissection
between pectoralis
major mus. and
breast tissue

C

D

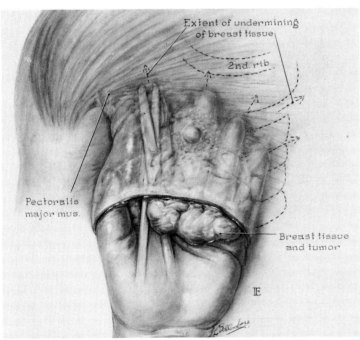

Extent of undermining
of breast tissue

2nd. rib

Pectoralis
major mus.

Breast tissue
and tumor

E

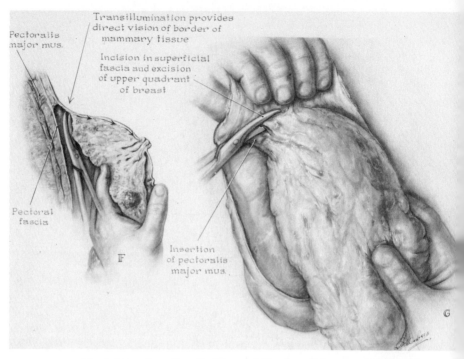

Fig. 4-4 (continued). **F.** After mobilization of the upper inner quadrant of the breast, a light is focused on the skin overlying the upper inner quadrant of the breast and the breast is detached from the fascia of the pectoralis major muscle and from the overlying skin. **G.** The skin of the breast is turned inside out and the breast tissue dissected away from the pectoralis major muscle under direct vision as well as away from the remaining skin and nipple. **H.** On the basis of the weight of the breast tissue resected, an appropriate silastic implant is selected and inserted into the pocket created between the fascia of the pectoralis major muscle and the skin of the breast. **I.** The silastic implant is positioned with the Teflon patch placed posteriorly against the fascia of the pectoralis major muscle, so that it will eventually be fixed in this position by adhesions. No sutures are employed.

flaps are quite thin and there is a 5 percent incidence of slough, necessitating subsequent skin grafts. Once these thin, widely mobilized skin flaps have healed, however, they are quite pliable and subsequent reconstruction with a Silastic implant is feasible. Wider excision of the skin of the breast avoids thin flaps and occasional skin slough, but this type of incision results in a wide scar which does not lend itself to subsequent reconstruction with a subcutaneous Silastic implant. Hultborn (26) and his associates have recently

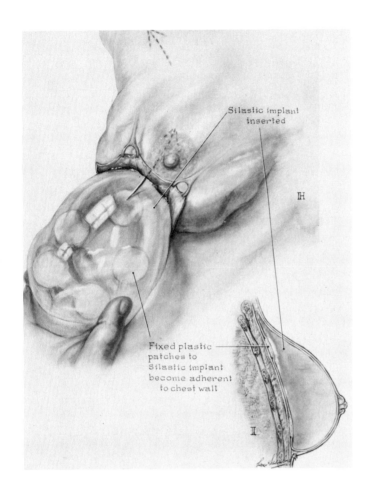

Silastic implant
inserted

IH

Fixed plastic
patches to
Silastic implant
become adherent
to chest wall

II

published an interesting study comparing the effectiveness of axillary lymph node dissection performed with preservation of the
pectoral muscles to an axillary dissection performed after excision of
the pectoral muscles. In this study one surgeon performed a modified
radical mastectomy and the operative specimen was submitted for
histologic study. A second surgeon then further dissected the axilla
after the pectoralis major and minor muscles were excised. This
study demonstrated that anywhere from three to ten additional

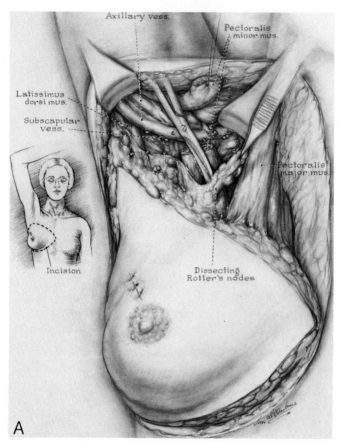

Fig. 4–5. **A.** The insert demonstrates the transverse incision and the mobility of the arm during the procedure. It is important to drape the arm in the sterile field so that it can be elevated during the axillary dissection. The large figure demonstrates the exposure of the axilla obtained after division of the pectoralis minor muscle and retraction

lymph nodes were removed by the surgeon who completed the excision of the pectoral muscles. The nodes which were not removed by the initial modified mastectomy were usually located in the apex of the axilla and in no instance did any of them contain metastatic tumor. Auchincloss (3) has demonstrated that the chances of survival are negligible if these apical lymph nodes contain metastatic carcinoma, and therefore excision of these nodes does not appear to add significantly to the patient's ultimate chance of survival.

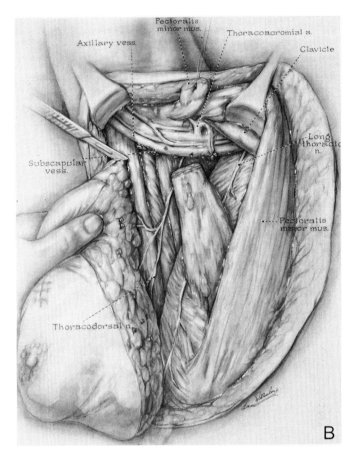

Of the pectoralis major muscle. The lymph nodes between the pectoralis major muscle and pectoralis minor muscles are excised. **B.** The completed axillary dissection. The pectoralis minor muscle is not reapproximated. The contents of the axilla following the axillary dissection are demonstrated.

The radical mastectomy described by Halsted excised the breast, the nipple, the underlying pectoralis major and minor muscles, and the contents of the axilla. This procedure is usually performed through a vertical incision, although it can be performed through a transverse incision. If large amounts of skin are removed, a skin graft is necessary for closure, but the majority of radical mastectomy incisions are now closed primarily, usually with moderate tension on the skin flaps. This procedure produces a cosmetic deformity characterized by a concavity of the chest wall below the clavicle, and of course, complete absence of the breast contour and nipple. A statistical evaluation of the complications of mastectomy has recently been published by Say and his associates (40). Skin-flap necrosis, serum collection beneath the skin flaps, wound infection, loss of skin grafts, and edema of the arm were the most common major complications. Lymphedema of the arm is the most serious long-term complication of a radical mastectomy and occurs in approximately 30 percent of the patients. In 10 percent of the patients, the lymphedema is severe enough to significantly limit motion of the arm and hand.

In the mid 1950s, Wagensteen (45) described the so-called superradical mastectomy which combined the Halsted radical mastectomy with excision of the supraclavicular nodes and excision of the internal mammary nodes. This operation was associated with considerably higher mortality rates than those associated with a radical mastectomy, and for this reason the procedure has never been widely accepted.

Urban (43) has also described an extended radical mastectomy which combined the Halsted radical mastectomy with excision of the internal mammary lymph nodes, but not with excision of the supraclavicular nodes. This procedure is commonly referred to as the Urban procedure. In addition to the standard Halsted mastectomy, the second, third, and fourth costal cartilages are excised with the lateral border of the sternum. The intercostal vessels and nodes are resected from the first through the fifth interspace. The resulting defect is either simply closed with the skin flap or closed with a free graft of fascia lata, a muscle flap, or marlex. Urban has been able to accomplish this procedure with the same mortality as that associated with a standard radical mastectomy. The functional and cosmetic deformity produced by the Urban procedure is similar to that produced by the radical mastectomy, as is the incidence of lymphedema of the arm.

Surgery is not the only ablative procedure which has been described in the management of breast cancer. Irradiation can be employed as the sole means of therapy or irradiation can be combined with quadrant excision, mastectomy, modified mastectomy, radical mastectomy, or the Urban procedure. When irradiation is employed as the primary means of therapy, the fields of irradiation usually include the breast, axillary lymph nodes, internal mammary lymph nodes, and supraclavicular lymph nodes. When irradiation is employed as an adjuvant, it can be administered either preoperatively or postoperatively. Irradiation produces a variety of changes in the skin, varying from slight erythema to ulceration. These acute inflammatory reactions usually subside after therapy has been completed, but residual shrinkage of the breast and radiation dermatitis, causing changes in the color of the skin, usually persists. Irradiation can also produce lymphedema of the arm secondary to ablation of the lymphatic channels in the axilla. Irradiation increases the incidence and severity of lymphedema occurring as the result of an axillary dissection. Irradiation can also produce a pneumonitis and subsequent fibrosis of the lung.

All of the ablative procedures described thus far are directed to the primary tumor and the regional lymph node-bearing areas, i.e., the axilla, the internal mammary lymph nodes, and the supraclavicular nodes. These procedures have no effect, of course, on circulating tumor cells or small foci of tumor cells which have implanted themselves in distant organs, such as the lung, bone, or liver. In an effort to kill or damage the circulating tumor cells or small foci of metastases, cytotoxic drugs (5-fluorouracil and thiotepa) have been administered at the time of mastectomy and for varying periods of time postoperatively. In addition to a possible cytotoxic effect on the tumor, these drugs are also toxic to the bone marrow and gastrointestinal tract.

Other systemic forms of therapy have also been evaluated. As early as 1900, some metastatic lesions of breast cancer were noted to disappear if the ovaries were removed from menstruating females. This type of breast cancer is referred to as hormone-dependent because the metastatic lesions appear to be dependent on the presence of estrogen. Within the past decade, oophorectomy has been combined with radical mastectomy, the rationale being to remove the primary tumor and to remove estrogen stimulation from any possible metastatic disease. The oophorectomy can be accomplished by either surgical excision or irradiation. The oophorectomy, of course, induces a menopause with its associated symptoms and thus compounds the emotional shock of losing a breast.

Summary of Results Obtained by Various Methods of Therapy. In spite of intensive investigation for the past fifty years, the treatment of breast cancer remains controversial. Innumerable retrospective studies have been published advocating one type of therapy or another, but firm conclusions cannot be made on the basis of these studies. In any type of valid clinical trial comparing one type of therapy to another, it is essential to estimate at least the clinical stage of disease prior to treatment and to randomize the patients into various treatment groups according to the estimated clinical stage of disease. Otherwise it is almost impossible to eliminate bias in the selection of treatment for individual patients. A few prospective trials which were conducted with the above principles in mind have been reported and some conclusions can be made on the basis of these reports. However, all of these reports can be criticized, even though they have employed pretreatment staging. All of the staging prior to treatment has been based on clinical findings alone. The results of these studies would have been more meaningful if the staging had included histologic findings as well, and thus compared the effect of different forms of therapy on specific histologic types and also on varying histologic grades of the tumor. In addition, most of the prospective studies have included far too many treatment variables and too few patients for accurate statistical analysis. All of these prospective clinical trials have recently been summarized by Fisher (17). In the following paragraphs these prospective trials are reviewed with appropriate comments.

Kaae and Johansen (28) have compared the results obtained following simple mastectomy combined with immediate postoperative irradiation to those obtained following an extended radical mastectomy including internal mammary node dissection. This study is difficult to evaluate, however, since the number of patients actually included in the randomized sample is quite small, thus affecting the statistical evaluation of the results. The five- and ten-year survival rates were the same whether the patient was treated by simple mastectomy and postoperative irradiation or by an extended radical mastectomy. The incidence of local recurrence was also the same. The incidence of lymphedema of the arm was increased in those patients who had an extended radical mastectomy.

Brinkley and Haybittle (6) compared the results obtained from simple mastectomy plus immediate postoperative irradiation to the results obtained after radical mastectomy either with or without postoperative irradiation. The source of the irradiation was a 250 Kv unit. All of the patients in the study had a palpable breast tumor and palpable but mobile axillary lymph nodes. There was no difference in the ten- to fifteen-year survival rates when results following simple mastectomy plus irradiation were compared to the results following radical mastectomy, either with or without postoperative irradiation. These results can be questioned because some of the patients undergoing simple mastectomy also had a variable number of low-lying axillary lymph nodes excised.

Bruce (7) has reported a similar trial, comparing the results obtained from simple mastectomy plus postoperative irradiation to those following a radical mastectomy. The patient population included patients with and without palpable axillary lymph nodes. All women under sixty also had a prophylactic oophorectomy. Those patients treated by radical mastectomy had a 10 percent greater survival rate compared to the group treated by simple mastectomy plus irradiation, but these results were not statistically significant.

Atkins (2) has reported a prospective study comparing the results obtained following quadrant excision and postoperative irradiation with those obtained following a radical mastectomy and postoperative irradiation in women over fifty years of age. Some of the patients also received a cytotoxic drug, thiotepa. The patients in the two treatment groups also received different types of irradiation. Those patients undergoing radical mastectomy received a relatively modest dose of orthovoltage irradiation postoperatively. The quadrant excision group of patients received a higher dose of irradiation via a linear accelerator. The five-year survival rates following quadrant excision and irradiation were similar to those obtained following radical mastectomy and irradiation, but only in those patients who had clinically negative axillary lymph nodes. In the presence of clinically positive axillary lymph nodes, Atkins reports that quadrant excision and irradiation were associated with considerably lower survival rates when compared to the survival rates obtained after radical mastectomy and irradiation. Rissanen (38) and Peters (35), in retrospective studies, have reported results comparing local excision and irradiation of the breast, axilla, supraclavicular area, and internal mammary nodal areas to those obtained following a radical mastectomy. There was no apparent difference in survival rates following either type of therapy.

A prospective study by Paterson and Russell (34) and a later report of the same study by Easson (12) demonstrated that postoperative irradiation does not add to the chance of survival following a radical mastectomy for breast cancer. It should be noted that this study employed orthovoltage irradiation. A similar study by Fisher (17) and his collaborators employing both orthovoltage and supervoltage irradiation equipment has also demonstrated no increase in survival rates following postoperative irradiation. These studies did demonstrate a lower incidence of local recurrence if postoperative irradiation was employed. Anderson (1), after surveying the literature and analyzing the results obtained in thousands of cases of breast cancer, has concluded that survival rates following postoperative irradiation are, if anything, reduced when compared with the results obtained after mastectomy alone.

Preoperative irradiation will also decrease the incidence of chest-wall recurrence; whether it adds anything to the chance of survival is controversial. Fletcher (19) reports that the age-adjusted, ten-year survival rates are better in patients treated with preoperative irradiation than in patients undergoing radical mastectomy without irradiation when axillary node status was similar. Lindgren's results (30) failed to demonstrate any increase in survival following the use of preoperative irradiation.

Ravdin's cooperative group (37), in a prospective study employing a relatively small number of patients, has demonstrated that a prophylactic oophorectomy in women less than fifty years of age does not increase their chance of subsequent survival after radical mastectomy for breast cancer. These figures differ somewhat from a study reported by Nissen-Meyer (32). Although Nissen-Meyer's study is controversial because a significant number of patients were excluded from the oophorectomy group on "ethical grounds," Nissen-Meyer's figures indicate that a prophylactic oophorectomy may be of benefit to postmenopausal women. There was no evidence that it was of benefit to premenopausal women. Cole (9) has also reported a study evaluating the effects of ovarian irradiation following a radical mastectomy in premenopausal women or in women within two years of the menopause. The resulting data fails to demonstrate any significant benefit from postoperative prophylactic castration by irradiation.

A few prospective studies have also evaluated prophylactic cytotoxic drugs as a means of increasing survival rates following the therapy of the primary tumor. The National Adjuvant Breast Project has evaluated the use of both an alkalating agent (thiotepa) and an anti-metabolite (5-FU) as a surgical adjuvant (15). These drugs were administered in the immediate postoperative periods, presumably to kill circulating tumor cells and/or foci of small metastases. The addition of these drugs as surgical adjuvants had no effect on survival rates. Similar studies have been reported from Scandinavia (33), employing cyclophosphamide in the immediate postoperative period. The authors of the Scandinavian study report a trend in favor of the use of cyclophosphamides as a surgical adjuvant, but their study is far from convincing because of the multiplicities of therapy directed toward the primary tumor.

Fisher and his associates (18) have recently described their experience with L-phenylalanine mustard as a surgical adjuvant in the management of patients with axillary lymph node metastases. All of the patients were treated by initial radical or modified radical mastectomy. If axillary lymph node metastases was present in the operative specimen the patients were randomized between the treated and control group. The patients undergoing treatment received 0.15 mg/kg of L-phenylalanine mustard per day for five consecutive days every six weeks. The control patients received a placebo. All patients were followed for at least eighteen months. Premenopausal women treated with L-phenylalanine mustard had a statistically significant longer disease-free interval than the control group. A similar trend was noted in postmenopausal women, but the initial results were not statistically significant and subsequent follow-up has failed to demonstrate any statistically significant increase in the disease-free interval. More recently the results in postmenopausal women have also become statistically significant. The L-phenylalanine mustard caused transient nausea and vomiting in some patients. Leukopenia was the only significant long-term complication. Of concern is the known increased incidence of leukemia in patients on long-term L-phenylalanine mustard. It should be emphasized, of course, that Fisher's data is preliminary. There is good evidence that the use of L-phenylalanine mustard will delay the detection of recurrence, there is no evidence at the present time that survival is prolonged. The results of this study are encouraging, however, and its progress should be carefully followed.

Bonadonna (5) has employed combinations of drugs as surgical adjuvant therapy. Three drugs have been utilized: cyclophosphamide, which is given by mouth, and intravenous injections of 5-fluorouracil and methotrexate. The drugs are administered in cyclical fashion at four-week intervals. Since combinations of cytotoxic drugs are more effective in the treatment of metastatic breast cancer than single drugs, the use of combination-drug therapy seems more promising than a single cytotoxic drug such as L-phenylalanine mustard. On the basis of preliminary data, there was a statistically significant lower incidence of treatment failures in patients on therapy compared to those patients who received a placebo. The progress of this study should also be carefully followed.

In summary, several definite statements can be made following review of these prospective clinical trials. Prophylactic irradiation of the ovaries or prophylactic oophorectomy in premenopausal women will not increase the chance of survival following a radical mastectomy. Preoperative irradiation may increase the chance of survival, but the clinical studies reported thus far are controversial. Partial mastectomy plus postoperative irradiation is as effective a means of treating breast cancer as radical mastectomy plus postoperative irradiation in women over fifty years of age with clinically negative axillary nodes. Partial mastectomy plus postoperative irradiation is associated with considerably poorer survival rates when compared to radical mastectomy plus postoperative irradiation in the presence of clinically positive axillary lymph nodes. There is probably no difference in survival rates when simple mastectomy plus postoperative irradiation is compared to a radical mastectomy. There is very little difference in survival rates following simple mastectomy and radical mastectomy in patients with clinically negative axillary lymph nodes. Long-term adjuvant chemotherapy, utilizing either L-phenylalanine mustard or a combination of cytoxan, methotrexate, and 5-fluorouracil does decrease the number of treatment failures within two years and may increase the chance of ultimate survival.

The management of inner quadrant and subaureloar lesions remains controversial. Urban (43) and Handley (25) have both demonstrated a high incidence of internal mammary node metastases in the presence of tumors beneath the nipple or in the inner quadrants of the breast. Urban's figures (44) indicate that some patients survive with both axillary and internal mammary nodal involvement, and these results have been confirmed by Livingston (31) and others. Handley's figures (25) indicate almost no chance of survival if the internal mammary nodes contain metastatic tumor. Lacour and his associates (29) have recently reported a clinical trial comparing the survival rates of patients undergoing radical mastectomy to those undergoing radical mastectomy plus internal mammary node dissection (Urban procedure). There was no difference in overall five-year survival rates between the two procedures. In one subgroup of patients, however, the Urban procedure was associated with an increased survival rate in comparison to the radical mastectomy. This group of patients had small medial quadrant lesions (T_1 and T_2) and histologic evidence of axillary lymph node metastases.

Treatment of the Individual Patient—Selecting the Optimal Means of Therapy on the Basis of the Clinical Assessment

There is no standard therapy or one operative procedure that is applicable to all patients with breast cancer. Therapy is based on the clinical assessment which will initially divide patients into two general categories: those patients with no clinical or radiographic evidence of distant metastases, and those patients with clinical or radiographic evidence of distant metastases. The latter patients are considered to be incurable, and their clinical management is discussed in the next chapter. In addition to those patients with clinical or radiographic evidence of distant metastases, certain other patients with advanced local disease are also considered to be incurable, because past experience has demonstrated that the great majority of them are dead of distant metastases within five years and that all of them are dead within ten years. These clinical signs of advanced local disease, which are almost invariably associated with occult systemic metastases, include patients with a primary tumor fixed to the chest wall, patients with satellite nodules in the skin of the breast, patients with palpable supraclavicular lymph nodes, patients with edema of the arm, and patients with histologic evidence of dermal lymphatic invasion.

Those patients with no clinical or radiographic evidence of distant metastases or evidence of advanced local disease can be treated by subcutaneous mastectomy and simultaneous or delayed silastic implant, by partial mastectomy, by simple mastectomy, by modified radical mastectomy (either with or without an internal mammary lymph node dissection), or by a radical mastectomy either with or without an internal mammary lymph node dissection. On the basis of the clinical assessment, which also includes a general assessment of any associated disease, one of these methods of therapy is selected. Associated disease of any severity generally precludes anything more extensive than a simple mastectomy, which usually can be performed under local anesthesia. If axillary lymph nodes are palpable, the axilla is irradiated if general anesthesia is contraindicated.

Subcutaneous mastectomy or partial mastectomy are not the procedures of choice in the majority of patients with breast cancer. It should be emphasized that these procedures are only considered if the patient is not a candidate for a total mastectomy because of associated disease or if the patient is anxious to preserve at least some of her breast. If there is no medical contraindication to a total mastectomy, or if conservation of the breast is not an issue, a total mastectomy is preferred. As previously noted, the primary objection to a partial mastectomy is the multifocal origin of a significant number of breast cancers. In spite of this high incidence of multifocal origin of breast cancer, Crile's (11) limited experience has demonstrated that at least an appreciable number of patients survive for prolonged periods of time after partial mastectomy, apparently because the microscopic foci of cancer in the other areas of the breast remain dormant and do not often become clinically apparent. The multifocal origin of breast cancer is not as potent an argument against a subcutaneous mastectomy as it is against a partial mastectomy, because a subcutaneous mastectomy removes 85 to 90 percent of the breast tissue and, therefore, most of the occult microscopic foci of tumor.

The management of the axillary lymph nodes is also controversial, although axillary lymph node dissection can be combined with a subcutaneous mastectomy or partial mastectomy. Since there are no clinical or radiographic methods which can provide an accurate assessment of the status of the axillary lymph nodes, many surgeons advocate routine excision of the axillary lymph nodes, even if no clinically suspicious lymphadenopathy is present. There is good evidence to support this position, since 30 percent of the patients with scirrhous duct carcinomas and clinically negative axillary lymph nodes who are subjected to radical mastectomy are found to have evidence of microscopic metastases in the axillary lymph nodes. In the presence of tumors of more favorable histologic patterns, such as a medullary carcinoma, colloid carcinoma, papillary carcinoma, or tubular carcinoma, however, the incidence of microscopic metastases in clinically negative nodes is probably considerably less than 30 percent, and a prophylactic axillary lymph node dissection is probably not necessary. In addition, the clinical studies reported by Atkins (2), Rissenen (38), and Crile (11) indicate that secondary treatment of axillary lymph nodes, i.e., an axillary dissection which is performed when the nodes become palpable, does not apparently lessen the chance of ultimate survival.

The choice between a subcutaneous mastectomy and a partial mastectomy is dependent upon a number of factors. The cosmetic result following a subcutaneous mastectomy is generally better than that obtained following partial mastectomy, particularly for lesions in the upper quadrants of the breast. The cosmetic result following a partial mastectomy for a lesion in the lower quadrants of the breast compares favorably with a subcutaneous mastectomy.

However, as previously noted, a subcutaneous mastectomy is a more extensive procedure than partial mastectomy and almost invariably has to be performed bilaterally, since it is not possible to remove the breast tissue from one breast and reconstruct it so that it even faintly resembles the opposite breast. Blood transfusions are occasionally necessary either during or following a subcutaneous mastectomy, and they are rarely necessary after a partial mastectomy. A partial mastectomy can usually be performed under local anesthesia, while a subcutaneous mastectomy invariably requires a general anesthesia.

The best indication for a subcutaneous mastectomy is lobular in situ carcinoma which is frequently a bilateral lesion. Subcutaneous mastectomies also appear to be reasonable procedures in patients with small (less than 2.0 cm) mobile tumors of favorable histologic pattern such as a medullary carcinoma, papillary carcinoma, comedocarcinoma, colloid carcinoma, or tubular carcinoma. In addition to this favorable histologic pattern, there should be no evidence of local skin or nipple retraction and no clinical evidence of axillary lymph node metastases. Subcutaneous mastectomies may also be reasonable procedures in patients with small scirrhous duct carcinomas of less than 2 cm in size. The scirrhous duct carcinomas should be of low histologic grade and there should be no evidence of necrosis within the tumor.

Partial mastectomies are primarily indicated in older women who are poor candidates for any type of more extensive operative procedure. These procedures may also be indicated in certain patients with low-grade tumors in the lower quadrants of the breast, i.e., patients with medullary carcinoma, colloid carcinoma, papillary carcinoma, or tubular carcinoma. In this situation there should also be no evidence of skin or nipple retraction and no clinical evidence of axillary lymph node metastases.

If the clinical data outlined above are not present, the patient is advised to have a modified radical mastectomy. A properly performed modified radical mastectomy removes all of the breast tissue but preserves skin flaps which will usually accept a silastic implant one to two years postoperatively, if the patient desires subsequent reconstruction. The procedure also removes the axillary lymph nodes, thus permitting histologic examination. At the present time histologic assessment of the axillary lymph nodes is the only means of accurately selecting patients for adjuvant chemotherapy. The majority of patients will accept a modified radical mastectomy, particularly if they are convinced that a careful clinical assessment has been performed and every effort made to determine the feasibility of a more conservative procedure. A smaller group of patients will, however, continue to refuse a mastectomy, even if axillary nodes are palpable. In this situation, partial mastectomy or subcutaneous mastectomy is combined with an axillary lymph node dissection. The patient should be aware that the procedure may not be associated with the same chance of survival as that obtained following a modified radical mastectomy.

As previously noted, a modified radical mastectomy is the procedure of choice in the majority of patients with breast cancer, i.e., those patients in the center of the spectrum of breast cancer. These patients have scirrhous duct carcinomas, the primary tumor is not fixed to the pectoral muscle, axillary lymph nodes may or may not be palpable, and there is no clinical or radiographic evidence of distant metastases. If the primary tumor is located in outer quadrants of the breast, a modified radical mastectomy is performed through a transverse incision. The only objections to a modified mastectomy compared to a radical mastectomy are the possibility of an increased incidence of local recurrence in the pectoral muscle and the slightly lesser chance of removing all of the axillary lymph nodes. Handley (25) has not seen a recurrence in the pectoral muscle following 800 consecutive cases treated by a modified radical mastectomy. The probable futility of removing apical axillary nodes has been previously discussed. If the tumor is located in the subaureolar area or in the inner quadrants of the breast, the decision as to the optimal means of therapy is more difficult. Currently available evidence indicates a high incidence of internal mammary node metastasis from lesions in the inner quadrants of the breast and from lesions in the subaureolar area. I don't see any rationale for an axillary dissection alone in this particular situation. If the axillary nodes are not involved, the procedure is not necessary. If the axillary nodes are involved, there is a very high incidence of internal mammary lymph node metastasis. Therefore, the internal mammary lymph nodes should be removed if your philosophy dictates removal of all lymph nodes with a reasonably good chance of metastatic involvement. In the presence of small inner quadrant lesions, or small lesions beneath the nipple (T_1 and T_2), an internal mammary node dissection combined with an axillary node dissection appears to be a reasonable procedure in patients under sixty-five years of age. The internal mammary node dissection can be performed either primarily or as a secondary procedure after the presence of axillary lymph node metastasis have been confirmed by histologic examination of the excised axillary lymph nodes. Internal mammary node dissections are technically more difficult than an axillary dissection alone, and the morbidity and mortality following these procedures is higher in inexperienced hands.

The patient with a so-called inflammatory carcinoma of the breast, with either erythema or ulceration of the skin overlying the tumor is most likely to die of breast cancer, even if there is no clinical or radiographic evidence of distant metastases. However, 5 to 15 percent of these patients will survive for five years, if these clinical findings are not associated with dermal lymphatic invasion. Irradiation is an acceptable means of therapy in these patients, and Guttman (23) has demonstrated that an appreciable number will live for five years if treated by irradiation alone. The selection of radical mastectomy versus primary irradiation therapy in patients with advanced local disease depends upon the clinical assessment, specifically the assessment of the growth rate of the tumor, its location, and its histologic grade. Patients with large indolent tumors which have been present for many years without evidence of distant metastases or fixed axillary lymph nodes are reasonable candidates for radical mastectomy, particularly if the tumor is of moderate or low histologic grade and is located predominately in the outer quadrants of the breast. Those patients with rapidly growing, high-grade tumors which are located in the inner quadrants of the breast are probably best managed by primary irradiation. These therapeutic decisions can be very difficult. Each case must be considered individually, and all aspects of the clinical assessment taken into consideration prior to any final decision.

The use of irradiation as a surgical adjuvant remains controversial. There is firm evidence from both prospective studies and retrospective analyses of large numbers of cases that postoperative irradiation has no effect on the survival of patients with breast cancer. Postoperative irradiation does decrease the incidence of local recurrence and therefore some investigators continue to advocate its use. In my opinion postoperative irradiation should not be employed. It does not seem worthwhile to irradiate one hundred patients if only 10 to 15 percent of them (i.e., that percentage of patients who may develop a local recurrence) will benefit from the postoperative irradiation. It is also conceivable, of course, that postoperative irradiation may be harmful in certain patients, since the incidence of liver metastases was increased in some of the patients receiving it, compared to those who were not irradiated. Furthermore, there is some question as to whether the majority of those patients who develop a local recurrence will receive any significant benefit from the irradiation. The majority of local recurrences, particularly those encountered after a total mastectomy, are due to blood-borne tumor cells implanting in the skin flaps, rather than residual tumor remaining after an inadequate excision (42). These local recurrences are simply the first manifestations of systemic recurrence and the local recurrences may respond to the modality of therapy selected for the systemic metastasis.

Preoperative irradiation may be of some benefit in reducing the incidence of local recurrence. However, there has been no conclusive evidence that preoperative irradiation prolongs survival, and until the controversy has been resolved, I would also not be in favor of the routine use of preoperative irradiation as a surgical adjuvant.

An increasing number of radiotherapists are advocating irradiation as the primary therapy for breast cancer (35, 36, 46). The advantages of radiotherapy as the sole means of therapy are obvious, it avoids an operative procedure and preserves the contour of the breast as well as the skin and nipple. The clinical evidence presented thus far indicates that survival rates following primary irradiation are similar, at least, to those following surgical excision. Definitive answers will only be available after prospective clinical trials have been performed, comparing excisional biopsy alone to excisional biopsy plus irradiation to mastectomy with or without axillary lymph node dissection. In my opinion, primary irradiation offers an alternate method of therapy, it does not offer a better method of therapy. If cosmesis is an issue with an individual patient, surgical excision and primary or delayed reconstruction probably offers a better cosmetic result than primary irradiation.

The previous discussion has probably covered 95 percent of the cases of breast carcinoma that will be encountered. A small percentage of unusual tumors is also encountered. The clinical management of these tumors is considered in the following paragraphs.

Cystosarcoma Phyllodes. These tumors present clinically as large, lobular masses which may have been present for a number of years. In spite of their large size, the overlying skin is usually not involved and the tumor mass has all the characteristics of a giant fibroadenoma, i.e., mobile, nontender, and not fixed to the overlying skin or surrounding breast tissue. There is no associated axillary lymphadenopathy. These large, bulky tumors are initially treated by excision. The operative specimen is examined histologically. If malignant, a wide field mastectomy is performed. Since a cystosarcoma phyllodes almost invariably metastasizes by blood-vessel invasion rather than by lymph node metastasis, an axillary lymph node dissection is not necessary.

Adenoid Cystic Carcinoma. These unusual breast cancers are similar to adenoid cystic carcinoma of salivary gland origin. A wide local excision will cure the patient in the great majority of cases, but every effort should be made to obtain a 2 to 3 cm margin of normal breast tissue around the tumor mass. Lymph node metastasis does not occur with these lesions. The most radical form of therapy therefore would be a simple mastectomy. Smaller tumors can be treated by a partial mastectomy or subcutaneous mastectomy.

Carcinoma in Children.   A form of breast carcinoma which is encountered in young children is described in Chapter 2. These cancers are locally excised with an adequate margin. Reconstruction is delayed until the opposite breast is fully developed.

Metaplastic Carcinomas.   These tumors are also briefly described in Chapter 2. Since lymph node metastases can occur, a modified radical mastectomy is advocated unless there is fixation to the chest wall. In the presence of fixation to the chest wall, a Halsted radical mastectomy is the procedure of choice.

Breast Carcinoma in the Male.   Carcinoma of the male breast accounts for approximately 1 percent of all breast carcinomas. The author has encountered one male with breast cancer who had two male siblings who also had breast carcinoma, and this increased familial incidence has also been reported by others. Some authors describe a poorer prognosis in male breast carcinomas compared with female breast carcinoma, but the lower survival rates in males are probably due to the fact that male breast carcinoma is encountered at a more advanced clinical stage. A high index of suspicion is necessary to detect early breast carcinoma in males. Gynecomastia is frequently encountered in elderly males, particularly cirrhotics and males on estrogen therapy for prostatic carcinoma. Gynecomastia can also be seen in association with certain carcinomas of the lung which produce a follicle-stimulating hormone. If there is no underlying cause for the gynecomastia, it should be excised for histologic study. The same general principles of management apply to breast carcinoma in males as have been described in the management of female breast carcinoma. The majority of patients are treated by a modified radical mastectomy, taking as much of the pectoralis major muscle as is necessary to remove the primary tumor with at least a 3 cm margin.

Carcinoma of the Breast Occurring during Pregnancy or Lactation.   Breast cancer is rare during pregnancy or lactation, occurring in approximately 2 to 3 patients per 1,000 pregnancies. The incidence varies with age and is slightly higher in an older population and considerably lower in a younger population. The majority of breast cancers occurring in pregnant or lactating women appear to be aggressive tumors which are frequently associated with axillary lymph node metastases and/or distant metastases. The generally poor prognosis of these tumors has been attributed to several different factors. The engorged breasts of the pregnant or lactating woman are more difficult to examine, and the patient or her physician does not detect a breast mass as easily as they might in a nonlactating breast. The diagnosis is thus delayed. Malignant tumors occurring during pregnancy may also be under increased hormonal stimulation, thus accounting for the seemingly more aggressive behavior. Treatment has been controversial primarily because no one surgeon or institution has had enough experience to come to any firm conclusions concerning optimal treatment. The following plan of management seems reasonable. Any suspicious mass detected during pregnancy or lactation should be biopsied under local anesthesia. It is important to proceed with the biopsy as soon as the mass is detected, thus avoiding any further delay in diagnosis if the mass proves to be malignant. If a diagnosis of a carcinoma is established, a modified radical mastectomy is performed. Termination of the pregnancy probably does not affect the patient's chances of survival. Some authors advise terminating the pregnancy if the breast cancer is associated with axillary lymph node metastases, but there is no statistical evidence to support this point of view. The prognosis is not hopeless, and in the absence of lymph node metastases survival rates as high as 60 percent have been reported. In the presence of lymph node metastases the chance of survival is considerably less.

Breast Cancer Presenting as a Palpable Axillary Lymph Node. Not all breast cancer presents as a palpable mass in the breast. Early tumors can be detected by mammography or xeroradiography, but unfortumately the first manifestation of some breast cancers is a palpable axillary lymph node. The palpable axillary lymph node may be associated with a breast cancer in the ipsilateral breast, although I have seen patients present with a palpable axillary lymph node which later proved to be from the contralateral breast. The tumor within the axillary lymph node may also be from another primary site, such as the lung or the gastrointestinal tract, or it may be the first manifestation of a lymphoma (10). If the patient with a palpable axillary lymph node has no evidence of a breast mass, a completely normal physical examination and a normal chest X-ray, a xeroradiogram is obtained. This study may reveal an occult breast cancer in either breast. If no evidence of an occult tumor can be found on xeroradiography, the axillary lymph node is excised. The presence of metastatic tumor compatable with a breast cancer is indication for removal of the ipsilateral breast and an axillary node dissection. In most cases the pathologist will find an occult primary tumor in the excised breast.

The Current Status of Surgical Adjuvants. In our opinion the drug regimens described by Fisher and Bonadonna should only be employed in selected patients, i.e., those patients with a significant chance of developing recurrence after initial therapy. At the present time histologic examination of the axillary lymph nodes is the only accurate method of predicting the chances of subsequent recurrence and, therefore, the indications for surgical adjuvant therapy. Women with no axillary lymph node metastases have a 75 percent chance of surviving for ten years without additional therapy, and the use of adjuvants in this group of patients is not indicated. Women with one to three axillary lymph nodes containing metastases, however, have a 60 percent chance of developing recurrence within ten years and therefore appear to be reasonable candidates for adjuvant chemotherapy, particularly if the chemotherapy is associated with little morbidity and almost no chance of mortality. Those women with four or more axillary lymph nodes containing metastatic tumor are excellent candidates for adjuvant chemotherapy, since they have at least an 85 percent chance of dying of metastatic tumor within ten years of initial therapy. In this group of patients, aggressive chemotherapy, associated with some morbidity and conceivably some slight mortality, seems warranted.

At the present time we are recommending the following types of adjuvant chemotherapy. All of our recommendations are based on the status of the axillary lymph nodes, thus reenforcing our preference for a modified radical mastectomy as the treatment of choice in most patients with breast cancer. The status of the axillary lymph nodes can, of course, only be determined if the pathologist has an opportunity to examine them.

In the absence of axillary lymph node metastases, we do not advise any adjuvant chemotherapy. If one to three axillary lymph nodes contain metastatic tumor, we advise L-phenylalanine mustard in premenopausal patients or patients within two years of the menopause. The drug is administered in a dosage of 0.15 mg/kg for five days every six weeks. The white blood cell count should be determined prior to each six-week cycle of therapy. If the white blood cell count falls below 3,000, the drug is not administered until the white blood cell count returns to normal. This drug regimen is maintained for two years. Other than transient nausea and vomiting, which can be controlled with anti-emetics, leukopenia is the only significant complication encountered thus far with this type of drug regimen. The vast majority of patients will note some irregularity in their menstrual cycles and 60 percent of the patients will not ovulate on this drug regimen.

Those patients with four or more axillary lymph nodes containing metastatic carcinoma and those postmenopausal women under age 70 with one to three axillary lymph nodes containing metastatic tumor are started on a drug regimen similar to that described by Bonadonna. Therapy is begun approximately one month after the modified radical mastectomy. Each cycle of therapy is repeated at twenty-eight-day intervals and consists of cyclophosphamide, 100 mg/m^2 by mouth on days one through fourteen of each cycle; 5-fluorouracil, 600 mg/mg^2 intravenously on days one and eight of each cycle; and methotrexate 40 mg/m^2 intravenously on day one and day eight of each cycle. Therapy is maintained for two years in the absence of significant toxicity. If the white blood cell count falls below 4,000, but is greater than 2,500, or if the platelets decrease to 75,000 to 100,000, 50 percent of the calculated dose of the drugs is given. If the white blood cell count falls below 2,500, or the platelet count falls below 75,000, all drugs are discontinued and only restarted when the white blood cell count and platelet count have returned to normal. Serum creatinine levels are obtained at monthly intervals and the methotrexate is discontinued if the serum creatinine rises to 1.5 mg% or above. If gross hematuria is detected, the cytoxan is discontinued until it subsides. All drugs are discontinued in the presence of oropharyngeal ulcers until these ulcers have healed. The majority of patients will not ovulate on this regimen, and approximately 30 percent of them will develop significant alopecia.

Follow-up Patients with No Axillary Lymph Node Metastases. As previously noted, those women with no evidence of axillary lymph node metastases are not candidates for adjuvant chemotherapy. Careful, periodic follow-up examinations, however, are of benefit, not only to detect a recurrence of the original tumor but also to detect a second primary tumor in the contralateral breast. The patients are initially followed at three-month intervals for the first two years following the treatment of the primary tumor and then at six-month intervals for the rest of their lives. The physical examination is repeated at each follow-up visit. A chest X-ray and xeroradiogram of the opposite breast are obtained at yearly intervals. In the absence of symptoms or positive physical findings, additional studies, such as a bone scan, brain scan, and liver scan, are not routinely performed. These scans supplemented by appropriate X-rays are obtained if there is any suggestion of metastatic disease by history and physical examination. Palpable evidence of recurrence is also promptly biopsied, not only to confirm the presence of recurrent tumor or metastases but also to obtain tumor for hormonal assay studies.

The problem of subsequent pregnancies in women with a history of breast cancer remains controversial. Most authorities advise avoiding pregnancy for at least two to three years after initial therapy. Subsequent pregnancy probably does not affect the ultimate chance of survival, but some authorities are opposed because an alteration in the hormonal milieu may activate occult metastases and thus shorten the symptom-free interval in certain patients. In general, patients with evidence of axillary lymph node metastases are advised to avoid pregnancy for at least five years. Those patients with no evidence of axillary lymph node metastases are advised to avoid pregnancy for at least two years following initial therapy. The management of patients with recurrent breast cancer is described in the following chapter. A second primary breast cancer in the contralateral breast is managed by the same principles that have been outlined in this chapter.

References

1. Anderson, J. M. 1973. A critique for the first treatment of carcinoma of the breast. *Surg. Gynec. Obstet.* 136:801.
2. Atkins, H., Hayward, J. L., and Klugman, D. J. 1972. Treatment of early breast cancer; a report after 10 years of a clinical trial. *Brit. Med. J.* 20:423.
3. Auchincloss, H. 1963. Significance of location and number of axillary metastases in carcinoma of the breast—a justification for a conservative operation. *Ann. Surg.* 158:37.
4. Bachman, A. L., and Sproul, E. E. 1955. Correlation of radiographic and autopsy findings in suspected metastases in the spine. *Bull. N.Y. Acd. Med.* 31:146.
5. Bonadonna, G., Brusamolino, E., Valagussa, P., Rossi, A., Brugnatelli, L., Brambilla, C., De Lena, M., Tacini, G., Bajetta, E., Musumeci, R., and Veronesi, U. 1976. Combination chemotherapy as an adjuvant treatment in operable breast cancer. *New Engl. J. Med.* 294:405.
6. Brinkley, D., and Haybittle, J. L. 1968. A 15-year follow-up study of patients treated for carcinoma of the breast. *Brit. J. Radiol.* 41:215.
7. Bruce, J. 1971. Operable cancer of the Breast. A controlled clinical trial. *Cancer* 28:1443.
8. Butcher, H. R., Jr., Seaman, W. B., Eckert, C., and Saltzstein, S. 1964. An assessment of radical mastectomy and postoperative irradiation therapy in the treatment of mammary cancer. *Cancer* 17:480.

9. Cole, N. P. 1968. Suppression of ovarian function in primary breast cancer. In: *Prognostic factors in breast cancer.* A. P. M. Forrest and P. B. Kunkler, eds. Edinburg, E. S. Livingstone, Ltd., p. 14. (From Proceedings of First Tenovus Symposium, Cardiff, 1967.)

10. Copeland, E. M., and McBride, C. M. 1973. Axillary metastases from unknown primary sites. *Ann. Surg.* 178:25.

11. Crile, G., Jr., Esselstyn, C. B., Jr., Hermann, R. E., and Hoerr, S. O. 1973. Partial mastectomy for cancer of the breast. *Surg. Gynec. Obstet.* 136:929.

12. Easson, E. C. 1968. Postoperative radiotherapy of breast cancer. In: *Prognostic factors in breast cancer.* A. P. M. Forrest and P. N. Kunkler, eds. Edinburg: E. S. Livingstone, Ltd., p. 146. (From Proceedings of First Tenovus Symposium, Cardiff, 1967.)

13. El-Domeiri, A. A. 1976. Role of preoperative bone scan in carcinoma of the breast. *Surg. Gynec. Obstet.* 142:722.

14. Ellis, D., and Teitelbaum, S. L. 1974. Inflammatory carcinoma of the breast. *Cancer* 33:1045.

15. Fisher, B., Ravdin, R. G., Ausman, R. K., Slack, N. H., Moore, G. E., Noer, R. J., and cooperative investigators. 1968. Surgical adjuvant chemotherapy in breast cancer, results of a decade of cooperative investigation. *Ann. Surg.* 168:337.

16. Fisher, B., Slack, N. H., Cavanaugh, P. J., et al. 1970. Postoperative radiotherapy in the treatment of breast cancer: Results of NSABP clinical trials. *Ann. Surg.* 172:711.

17. Fisher, B. 1973. Cooperative clinical trials in primary breast cancer, a critical appraisal. *Cancer* 31:1271.

18. Fisher, B., Carbon, P., Economou, S. G., Frelick, R., Glass, A., Lerner, H., Redmond, C., Zelen, M., Band, P., Katrych, D. A., Wolmark, N., and Fisher, E. R. 1975. L-phenylalanine mustard (L-PAM) in the management of primary breast cancer. *New Engl. J. Med.* 292:117.

19. Fletcher, G. H., et al. 1968. Evaluation of irradiation of the peripheral lymphatics in conjunction with radical mastectomy for cancer of the breast. *Cancer* 21:791.

20. Gallagher, H. S., and Martin, J. E. 1969. Early phases in the development of breast cancer. *Cancer* 24:1170.

21. Galasko, C. S. B., Westerman, B., Li, J., Sellwood, R. A., and Burn, J. I. 1968. Use of the gamma camera for early detection of osseous metastases from mammary cancer. *Brit. J. Surg.* 55:613.

22. Grace, J. T., and Dao, T. L. 1959. Etiology of inflammatory reaction in breast carcinoma. *Surg. Forum* 9:611.

23. Guttman, R. 1967. Radiotherapy in locally advanced cancer of the breast. *Cancer* 20:1046.

24. Halsted, W. S. 1894. Results of operation for cure of cancer of breast performed at Johns Hopkins Hospital from January 1889–January, 1894. *Ann. Surg.* 20:497.

25. Handley, R. S. 1969. A surgeon's view of the spread of breast cancer. *Cancer* 24:1231.

26. Hultborn, A., Hulten, L., Roos, B., Rosencrantz, M., Rosengren, B., and Ahren, C. 1974. Effectiveness of axillary lymph node dissection in modified radical mastectomy with preservation of pectoral muscles. *Ann. Surg.* 179:269.

27. Jaffe, H. L. 1958. *Tumors and tumorous conditions of bones and joints.* Philadelphia.

28. Kaae, S., and Johansen, H. 1968. Simple versus radical mastectomy in primary breast cancer. In: *Prognostic factors in breast cancer.* A. P. M. Forrest and P. B. Kunkler, eds. Edinburgh: E. D. Livingstone, Ltd., p. 93.

29. Lacour, J., Bucalossi, P., Cacers, E., et al. 1976. Radical mastectomy versus radical mastectomy plus internal mammary dissection. *Cancer* 37:206.

30. Lindgren, M., Borgstrom, S., and Landberg, T. 1968. Preoperative radiotherapy in operable breast cancer. In: *Prognostic factors in breast cancer.* A. P. M. Forrest and P. B. Kunkler, eds. Edinburg: E. D. Livingstone, Ltd., p. 103.

31. Livingston, S. F., and Arlen, M. 1974. The entended extrapleural radical mastectomy, *Ann. Surg.* 179:260.
32. Nissen-Meyer, R. 1965. Castration as part of the primary treatment for operable female breast cancer. *ACTA Radiol. Suppl.* 249:1.
33. Nissen-Meyer, R., Kjellgren, K., and Mansson, B. 1971. Preliminary report from the Scandinavian Adjuvant Chemotherapy Study, *Cancer chemother. rep.* 55:561.
34. Paterson, R., and Russell, M. H. 1959. Clinical trials of malignant disease—III. breast cancer; evaluation of postoperative radiotherapy. *J. Fac. Radiol.* 10:175.
35. Peters, M. V. 1967. Wedge resection and irradiation: An effective treatment in early breast cancer. *JAMA* 200:144.
36. Prosnitz, L. R., Goldenberg, I. S. 1975. Radiation therapy as primary treatment for early stage carcinoma of the breast. *Cancer* 35:1587.
37. Ravdin, R. G., Lewison, E. F., Slack, N. H., Dao, T. L., Gardner, B., State, D., and Fisher, B. 1970. Results of a clinical trial concerning the worth of prophylactic oophorectomy for breast carcinoma. *Surg. Gynec. Obstet.* 131:1055.
38. Rissanen, P. M. 1969. A comparison of conservative and radical surgery combined with radiotherapy in the treatment of Stage I carcinoma of the breast. *Brit. J. Radiol.* 42:423.
39. Rosen, P. P., Fracchia, A. A., Urban, J. A., Schottenfeld, D., and Robbins, G. F. 1975. "Residual" mammary carcinoma following simulated partial mastectomy. *Cancer* 35:739.
40. Say, C. C., and Donegan, W. 1974. A biostatistical evaluation of complications from mastectomy. *Surg. Gynec. Obstet.* 138:370.
41. Shah, J. P., Rosen, P. P., and Robbins, G. F. 1973. Pitfalls of local excision in the treatment of carcinoma of the breast. *Surg. Gynec. Obstet.* 136:721.
42. Spratt, J. S. L. 1967. Locally recurrent cancer after radical mastectomy. *Cancer* 20:1051.
43. Urban, J. A. 1952. Radical mastectomy in continuity with En block resection of the internal mammary lymph node chain. *Cancer* 5:992.
44. Urban, J. A., and Castro, E. B. 1971. Selecting variations in the extent of surgical procedures for breast cancer. *Cancer* 28:1615.
45. Wagensteen, O. H. 1952. Super-radical operation for breast cancer in the patient with lymph node involvement. *Proc. 2nd Nat. Cancer Congress*, p. 230.
46. Weber, E. 1975. Radiation as primary treatment for local control of breast carcinoma. *JAMA* 234:608.

5. THE CLINICAL MANAGEMENT OF METASTATIC OR RECURRENT BREAST CANCER

Martin D. Abeloff and R. Robinson Baker

Eighty-eight thousand new cases of carcinoma of the female breast will occur in the United States in 1976. Approximately 50 percent of these patients are cured. The remaining patients, approximately 44,000 women per year, will develop evidence of recurrence. In the majority of cases the recurrence means distant metastases; in a smaller percentage of cases, a local lesion either on the chest wall or in the regional lymph nodes is the only manifestation of recurrence. Metastatic or recurrent breast cancer varies dramatically in its clinical course. Most patients with metastatic breast cancer should be promptly treated to relieve or prevent progressively severe symptoms. A few patients with metastatic breast cancer, however, will live for years without symptoms and require no therapy. It is important, therefore, in the clinical management of patients with recurrent breast cancer to assess the tempo of the metastatic disease that is present and to make therapeutic decisions which reflect the rate of progression of the disease. In some cases systemic treatment with cytotoxic drugs is indicated immediately; in other cases an isolated metastasis may respond to irradiation, and no other treatment is necessary.

Prior to any discussion of the treatment modalities that are available, the natural history of breast cancer will be briefly reviewed and various discriminant clinical factors which are meaningful in the prediction of subsequent behavior will be described. The survival time of patients with untreated breast cancer varies from six months to nineteen years. Approximately 20 percent of patients with untreated breast cancer survive for five years. Of those potentially curable patients who are treated by a radical mastectomy and are found to have no evidence of axillary lymph node metastases, 80 percent will survive five years. If four or more axillary lymph nodes contain metastatic tumor, the chance of five-year survival falls to 15 percent (18). The pattern of recurrence varies considerably. Four to 5 percent of patients with recurrent breast cancer will develop an isolated recurrence on the chest wall or in the axillary, supraclavicular, or internal mammary lymph nodes. In a much larger percentage of patients, the first manifestation of metastases will be at a distant site or the local recurrence and distant metastases will appear synchronously. The most common site of initial metastases is the skeletal system (osseous recurrence), specifically the ribs and spine. The respiratory system is the second most common site of clinically diagnosed metastases. Fifty to 60 percent of metastases will become apparent within three years of initial therapy, 85 percent within five years, and 98 percent within ten years. Once a metastasis has been detected 50 percent of the patients will be dead within eight months, and 80 percent will be dead within twenty-four months (18).

Clinical Assessment

The clinical assessment is designed to determine the cause of symptoms and their severity, the menopausal status of the patient and the hormone dependency of the tumor, the location of dominant metastatic disease and the rate of its progression.

History. The initial history focuses on the details of the diagnosis and therapy of the primary tumor. The type of operative procedure is determined and the histologic sections of the primary tumor and available lymph nodes are reviewed. Specific inquiries are made regarding the use of adjuvants to the surgical procedure, such as irradiation, endocrine ablative procedures, or cytotoxic drugs. The disease-free interval, i.e., that period of time between the primary therapy and the first indication of recurrence or metastases, is calculated. Precise information regarding the patient's menstrual history is essential for decisions regarding therapy of the recurrent cancer.

The type and severity of symptoms are recorded and the degree of disability produced by the metastatic disease is estimated. The history of the patient's current problems is taken in the context of a thorough general review of the past medical history.

Physical Examination.   Local recurrence in the skin flaps following a mastectomy can present initially as tiny erythematous lesions which look quite innocuous. If their etiology is in doubt, a punch biopsy of the lesion can be obtained. Recurrent breast cancer on the chest wall is usually more obvious and is characterized by a hard, fixed mass. Metastases can also occur in the opposite breast, but this is infrequent. Both the ipsilateral and contralateral axillae and supraclavicular fossae are examined for evidence of metastatic disease. Nodes in the internal mammary chain may be involved, and as these nodes enlarge, they may project through the intercostal spaces. On examination of the chest one looks for evidence of a pleural effusion or consolidation of the underlying lung parenchyma. The abdomen is examined for evidence of hepatomegaly, peritoneal implants, or ascites. All neurologic deficits are recorded. A careful search should be made for signs of spinal cord compression, including weakness in the extremities, changes in deep-tendon reflexes, and sensory deficits.

Laboratory Studies.   Routine blood studies, including a hematocrit, white blood cell count, and platelet count, are obtained on all patients. Anemia or pancytopenia can be due to marrow replacement by metastatic tumor or to marrow depression by previous therapeutic maneuvers. A serum calcium is determined, since hypercalcemia occurs in 10 to 20 percent of patients with metastatic breast cancer. Hypercalcemia generally is associated with skeletal lytic metastases and can also be precipitated by therapy with estrogens, androgens, and progestins. The serum alkaline phosphatase may be elevated in the presence of liver or bone metastases. If elevated, the serum alkaline phosphatase can often serve as an indicator of the response of metastatic disease to treatment. In view of the fact that most patients will eventually become candidates for chemotherapy, liver and renal function studies are obtained, since many of the cytotoxic drugs are excreted by the liver or kidney.

A biochemical marker which reflected the clinical or subclinical tumor burden of the patient would be most helpful in following the course of metastatic breast cancer. Carcinoembryonic antigen (CEA), a glycoprotein first described by Gold and Freedman (24), has been useful in monitoring the course of colon carcinoma. CEA was originally thought to be endodermally derived; but elevated serum CEA levels have now been described in a variety of nondigestive tract tumors as well as nonmalignant disorders, such as inflammatory bowel disease, metabolic disorders, and pulmonary disease (14). Recent studies have demonstrated elevation of serum CEA in 74 to 79 percent of patients with metastatic breast carcinoma (48, 53). In a small number of patients, the serial CEA values correlated with the response to therapy of the metastatic breast carcinoma. Clinical trials are continuing with CEA and batteries of biologic markers (53) which may provide objective serologic evidence of tumor progression or regression prior to the time that such changes are clinically evident.

Radiographic Studies. Radiographic studies are designed to document the presence of metastases which are suggested by the history and physical examination. In most situations these radiographic studies include a chest X-ray, xeroradiography of the remaining breast, a bone scan supplemented by appropriate X-rays and tomograms, a liver scan, and a brain scan. In addition, radiographic studies also provide a means of detecting occult asymptomatic metastases. A bone scan is an effective technique for detecting occult osseous lesions in asymptomatic patients, but the brain scan is rarely positive in the absence of neurologic signs or symptoms. Liver scan is recommended in the presence of hepatomegaly or abnormal liver function tests, but not as a routine screening test.

Although bone scans are far more sensitive detectors of skeletal metastases than bone roentgenograms, the radioisotope studies do not clearly differentiate between metastatic disease and other causes of increased concentration of isotope, such as osteoarthritis. Bone scans also do not provide practical information regarding the degree of destruction of the involved bones. Skeletal roentgenograms, either plain X-rays and/or tomograms, should, therefore, be obtained to confirm the presence of a metastatic lesion and also to follow the architectural integrity of the involved bones. Careful X-ray monitoring of skeletal lesions can lead to initiation of radiation therapy and/or orthopedic procedures before pathologic fractures occur.

Studies of Hormonal Status. An empirical observation was made in the latter part of the nineteenth century that certain patients with metastatic breast cancer were effectively palliated by an oophorectomy, i.e., symptoms were relieved and there was objective evidence of regression of the tumor (5). This initial observation was confirmed by numerous studies which have demonstrated that 20 to

50 percent of premenopausal women with metastatic breast cancer will show both subjective and objective evidence of improvement following an oophorectomy (34, 36). It has also been clearly established that women who are four or more years postmenopausal have a 20 to 40 percent response rate to additive estrogen therapy (13, 33).

Hormonal therapy is thus of benefit to some patients, but until recently there was no adequate method of predicting a response. Vaginal cytology will provide a reasonably accurate estimate of the levels of endogenous estrogen production, in that estrogen stimulates the vaginal mucosa and women with significant estrogen secretion will have a cornified vaginal epithelium. However, this type of study provides no information concerning the hormone dependency of the tumor. In the past decade, laboratory procedures have been developed which provide an improved means of predicting the chances of response to oophorectomy and other endocrine ablative or additive procedures. Folca et al. reported in 1961 that tritium-labeled hexestrol was taken up to a greater extent by tumors from patients with breast cancer who later responded to ablative endocrine surgery than by tumors from nonresponsive patients (20). A number of investigators have subsequently demonstrated that certain breast cancers contain cytoplasmic proteins (estrogen receptors or estrogen-binding proteins) which are capable of binding estradiol (31, 38, 49, 51). The initial studies were qualitative, but more recently quantitative methods of measuring the number of specific estradiol binding sites per unit of tissue have been developed (44).

These studies have indicated that approximately 30 percent of tumors from premenopausal women contain measurable levels of estrogen receptors, while 68 percent of postmenopausal women have primary tumors in which estrogen-binding protein can be identified (55). Clinical studies which have correlated response to hormone therapy with the presence or absence of estrogen receptors have demonstrated that if the estrogen receptors are present in the cytoplasm of the tumor cells there is at least a 50 percent chance of the patient responding to either ablative or additive endocrine therapy. In the absence of estrogen receptors, there is very little chance of the patient responding to endocrine therapy (45). At the present time, the estrogen receptor assay would appear to be most useful for identifying those patients who have virtually no chance of responding to hormonal therapy. Recently, Horwitz, McGuire, and colleagues (30) have described the presence of a protein in certain breast cancer cells which specifically binds progesterone (progesterone receptors). These progesterone receptors were found in 56 percent of those tumors with estrogen receptors, but were absent in tumors without estrogen receptors. Responses to endocrine therapy were only obtained in those patients with progesterone receptors. If this preliminary data is supported by additional clinical trials, the use of progesterone receptors may greatly refine our ability to predict response to additive or ablative endocrine therapy.

Since the commercially available quantitative methods of measuring estrogen-binding protein require fairly large amounts of tissue (i.e., 1 gram), and tumor tissue may not be accessible to biopsy at the time of the development of recurrent or metastatic disease, it is important that the estrogen receptor assay be performed with tissue obtained from primary breast cancers. If the patient subsequently develops clinical evidence of metastases, the presence or absence of estrogen-binding protein will be known, and future therapy can be planned accordingly. If the primary tumor was not assayed for receptors, then biopsies of metastatic lesions should be obtained for receptor assays.

Summary of Clinical Assessment. On the basis of the history, physical examination, laboratory studies, and radiographic studies, the predominant site of recurrence is characterized as nodal or soft tissue, osseous, or visceral. The predominant site of recurrence, the extent of the metastatic disease (local or disseminated), the disease-free interval, the age of the patient are helpful in predicting the clinical course of the patient and the need for systemic therapy. The premenopausal patient with a short disease-free interval and diffuse metastases in the lung, liver, or central nervous system has a very poor prognosis and requires systemic therapy if effective palliation is to be achieved. In contrast, the postmenopausal patient with a long disease-free interval and a local soft tissue or osseous recurrence has a more favorable prognosis and is likely to do well on either local or systemic therapies. The majority of the patients fall into the spectrum somewhere between these two extremes and will require systemic therapy shortly after the diagnosis of metastatic disease has been established. The choice of hormonal therapy versus chemotherapy is made with the knowledge of menstrual history, vaginal cytology, and estrogen receptor assay.

Treatment—General Principles

Unlike most solid tumors, breast cancer responds to a variety of therapeutic modalities, including endocrine ablative procedures, additive endocrine therapy, cytotoxic chemotherapy, and radiation therapy. Although current therapies for metastatic disease do not result in cure, the responders to systemic therapy do achieve relief of symptoms and prolongation of life.

In comparing the effectiveness of antitumor therapies, it is essential to establish rigid criteria for defining response. Response as used in this chapter is defined by the criteria of the Cooperative Breast Cancer Group (12). A partial response indicates a 50 percent decrease in size of at least 50 percent of the measurable lesions, while the remaining lesions are unchanged and no new lesions appear. The objective changes must be accompanied by subjective improvement. Complete response refers to the complete disappearance of all measurable lesions and a return to the asymptomatic state. In osteolytic lesions, roentgenographic evidence of healing is required. Osteoblastic lesions and pleural effusions are not considered measurable disease. The disease is considered progressive if there is objective increase in any lesion with or without subjective improvement.

The choice of an appropriate therapeutic modality is based on the clinical assessment of the patient and a thorough understanding of the different types of treatment. A logical diagnostic and therapeutic plan is essential from the time of initial diagnosis of metastatic disease if optimal results are to be achieved with our treatment modalities. In this section, the general principles of the major forms of therapy will be reviewed. Specific treatment plans based on these principles will be discussed in the following section.

Castration. In 1896, Sir George Beatson reported the remission of advanced breast cancer in two women on whom he had performed bilateral oophorectomy (5). Since that time, castration has been shown to result in objective responses in 20 to 50 percent of premenopausal women with metastatic breast cancer (36). The duration of response averages eight to twelve months and responders survive longer than nonresponders. Oophorectomy is generally not efficacious in postmenopausal women. It has also been well established that prophylactic castration (35) does not increase survival in breast cancer.

Castration can be accomplished either by surgical excision or irradiation. Surgical excision removes the source of estrogen produced by the ovaries immediately and also provides an opportunity to assess the extent of intraperitoneal disease, particularly liver metastases. However, the antitumor effect of castration may not become apparent for eight to 12 weeks following the removal of the ovaries. Irradiation castration results in a more gradual diminishing of ovarian function than surgical oophorectomy and, therefore, the therapeutic response may be proportionately delayed. In addition, there is a risk of incomplete ablation of ovarian function by radiotherapy, particularly in young women. Candidates for castration are, therefore, advised to have surgical oophorectomy. If the patient refuses surgery or surgical excision is contraindicated because of associated disease, irradiation castration is an acceptable alternative.

Castration is not only an effective therapeutic modality in the premenopausal patient with metastatic disease but it also provides an estimate of the likelihood of response to subsequent endocrine therapy. Patients who achieve an objective response following castration have approximately a 50 percent response rate to secondary ablative procedures (i.e., hypophysectomy or adrenalectomy), while those who do not respond to castration have a low response rate (generally less than 20 percent) to subsequent endocrine therapy (21).

Estrogen and Androgen Therapy. In postmenopausal women with metastatic disease, additive estrogen therapy occupies a position similar to that of castration in the therapeutic strategy of premenopausal women. Estrogens result in a response rate of 20 to 40 percent (36). The response rate to estrogens is generally higher in predominately soft tissue and nodal disease than in osseous and visceral metastases. The majority of patients who are going to respond to estrogens will show some evidence of tumor regression within eight weeks of initiation of therapy. The mean duration of response has been reported to be as long as 20+ months and the responders to estrogens do survive longer than the nonresponders (33). The most commonly used estrogenic hormones are diethylstilbestrol (5 mgm three times a day) and ethinyl estradiol (0.5-1.0 mgm three times a day). Although the estrogen preparations are generally well tolerated by the patient, these hormones can cause a myriad of side effects. The adverse effects can include anorexia, nausea, vomiting, fluid retention and congestive heart failure, urinary urgency and incontinence, engorgement of the remaining breast and pigmentation of the aureola, and uterine bleeding. These effects of estrogen can be most distressing to the patient, but the most serious toxicity of estrogen therapy is the induction of hypercalcemia. Estrogen-induced hypercalcemia generally occurs within one to two months of the initiation of estrogen therapy. The onset of symptoms (nausea, vomiting, constipation, polyuria, polydipsia, lethargy, and a variety of neurologic disorders) is often insidious, and these symptoms may be erroneously attributed to other effects of the underlying malignancy. The hallmark of therapy of estrogen-induced hypercalcemia is discontinuation of the estrogens and vigorous hydration. Mithramycin therapy is a rapid and safe way of temporarily controlling the hypercalcemia (40).

The role of androgens in the therapeutic strategy of metastatic breast cancer is unclear. Comparative trials have demonstrated that androgens have a significantly lesser response rate than estrogens (13, 33). Osseous metastases do appear to respond equally well to estrogens and androgens. Androgens are largely reserved for post-menopausal women. In premenopausal women, androgen therapy is generally restricted to selected patients who have failed to respond to castration.

In addition to many of the side effects caused by estrogens, androgens also can cause virilization and hepatic dysfunction. These anabolic steroids have been shown to provide symptomatic improvement (increase in appetite and weight, general sense of well being) even in the face of objective progression of the disease.

A variety of androgenic preparations are available, and the antitumor effects of these agents are similar. Fluoxymesterone (Halotestin) and calusterone (Methosarb) are oral preparations and are administered in doses of 10 mg twice a day and 50 mg four times a day, respectively. Testosterone propionate and Testolactone (Teslac) are administered in doses of 100 mg intramuscularly three times a week. Testosterone propionate and fluoxymesterone are reported to have more virilizing effects than calusterone. Testolactone is devoid of virilizing effects, but it is not as effective an antitumor agent as the other testosterone derivatives.

Estrogens and androgens are, therefore, the mainstay of additive hormonal therapy. However, the use of massive doses of progestins have been reported to be effective in approximately 20 percent of patients (3). These preliminary trials require confirmation before these agents are included in the therapeutic armamentarium of metastatic breast cancer.

Secondary Ablative Therapy. The hormonal dependency of certain breast cancers can be further exploited by bilateral adrenalectomy or hypophysectomy. These major operative procedures are generally regarded as secondary endocrine therapy in that they are reserved for patients who have responded to castration or hormonal additive therapy and have subsequently relapsed.

The overall response rates to adrenalectomy and hypophysectomy are not significantly different (22). MacDonald reported a 28 percent regression rate in 690 patients who underwent adrenalectomy and a 33 percent response rate in 340 patients who were treated with hypophysectomy (43). As is true in the other therapeutic approaches to breast cancer, the responders not only achieved relief of symptoms but survived longer than nonresponders. The responders to adrenalectomy and hypophysectomy had mean survivals of twenty-four and twenty-three months respectively. Because of the operative morbidity and mortality (5 percent), the limited response rate and survival, it is important to carefully select patients for these procedures. Patients who have responded favorably to previous castration or estrogen therapy are most likely to achieve response from secondary procedures. A negative estrogen receptor test indicates that the patient is unlikely to benefit from adrenalectomy or hypophysectomy. Patients who have widespread visceral metastases are generally not good operative risks and are not likely to respond to these procedures.

The response and mortality rates of the two operations are essentially the same. The choice of procedure must largely depend on the skill of the surgeon and the general medical status of the patient. With improvement in the technique of transphenoidal hypophysectomy, pituitary ablation involves shorter hospitalization and less morbidity than adrenalectomy and is becoming the operation of choice for the majority of patients (10). In the hands of an experienced operator, a transphenoidal hypophysectomy can be accomplished by a transnasal approach. Following such a procedure the patient is maintained on 37.5 mgm of cortisone acetate a day and 2 grains of dessicated thyroid or its equivalent of synthetic preparations. Posterior pituitary powder is usually necessary to manage the induced diabetes insipidus. Complications include: meningitis, rhinorrhea, visual impairment, and an impairment of taste.

Bilateral adrenalectomy can be performed through either an anterior transperitoneal approach or posteriorly through the bed of the resected twelfth rib. Mortality rates are equivalent to those of a hypophysectomy. Complications include postoperative bleeding and the sequelae of any major intra-abdominal procedure. Postoperatively the patients are maintained on cortisone acetate and fluorohydrocortisone to replace the mineralocorticoid activity of the adrenal glands.

The indications for these secondary ablative procedures remain controversial, particularly since the advent of combination drug therapy. Although some investigators recommend adrenalectomy as initial therapy for metastatic disease (54), hypophysectomy and adrenalectomy are generally reserved for patients who have had previous response to hormonal therapy and have predominantly soft tissue, nodal, or osseous metastases.

Since many patients with metastatic breast cancer are poor risks for any operative procedure, there has also been considerable interest in medical ablation of adrenal steroidogenesis. "Medical adrenalectomy" using aminoglutethemide (a direct inhibitor of adrenal steroid synthesis) has been reported to produce objective remissions in far advanced breast cancer (28) and is undergoing further trials (41).

Chemotherapy. It has been recognized for many years that metastatic breast cancer is responsive to drugs from each of the major categories of cytotoxic chemotherapeutic agents (Table 5-1). However, the responses to these single agents have generally been incomplete and the duration of responses has been brief.

In 1963, Greenspan published a 60 percent response rate in the treatment of metastatic breast cancer with methotrexate and thio-TEPA (an alkylating agent) (26). Greenspan subsequently reported an 81 percent response rate with a five-drug combination (27). Interest in combination chemotherapy in breast cancer remained relatively dormant, but received a major boost by the successful application of multi-drug therapy in acute leukemia (23), Hodgkin's disease (17), and non-Hodgkin's lymphoma (29). Cooper's report in 1969 of a 90 percent regression rate in breast cancer with cyclophosphamide, 5-fluorouracil, methotrexate, vincristine, and prednisone (11) inaugurated an era of great activity in the chemotherapy of breast cancer.

Table 5-1.
Effective Cytotoxic Drugs in Metastatic Breast Cancer

Category of cytotoxic agents	Specific drug	Objective response rate	References
Antibiotic	Adriamycin	48%	25
Alkylating agent	Cyclophosphamide	35%	8
Antimetabolite	Methotrexate	41%	8
Antimetabolite	5-Fluorouracil	23%	2
Vinca alkaloid	Vincristine	20%	8
Corticosteroid	Prednisone	18%	37

Cyclophosphamide, methotrexate, 5-fluorouracil, vincristine, and prednisone have subsequently been employed in a variety of combinations. Carter has reviewed the literature on these modifications of the Cooper regimen and has noted an average response rate of 48 percent, with a range of 29 percent to 70 percent (9). Differences in intensity of treatment, patient selection, criteria for responses, and data reporting account for the broad range of responses.

Following the identification of the anthracycline antibiotic, Adriamycin, as perhaps the most single effective agent in metastatic breast cancer (6, 9), a number of regimens combining Adriamycin with an alkylating agent and/or antimetabolite have been devised. Jones and his co-workers have reported a response rate of 80 percent with Adriamycin and cyclophosphamide (32), and Blumenschein and colleagues have noted a 72 percent response rate with Adriamycin, cyclophosphamide, and 5-fluorouracil (7). The preliminary reports of these newer combinations are encouraging, but it must be emphasized that the most effective combination of drugs has not been established. In fact, it has not been unequivocally demonstrated that combination chemotherapy results in better survival than single agents used in a sequential fashion (4). However, it is clear that a number of chemotherapy programs can result in a response rate of 45 percent or greater in patients with far advanced breast cancer (Table 5-2). Responders generally enjoy quantitatively and qualitatively better survival than nonresponders.

An example of a combination chemotherapy regimen that has resulted in a 46 percent response rate (39) in the Johns Hopkins Breast Clinic is outlined in Table 5-3. It is now generally agreed that if a complete or partial remission is achieved with such a chemother-

Table 5-2.
Combination Chemotherapy for Metastatic Breast Cancer

Combinations	Objective response rate	Reference
Cy, Mtx, 5-Fu, Vcr, Pred	46%	39
Cy, Mtx, 5-FU	52%	50
Adria, Vcr	48%	16
Adria, Cy	80%	32
Adria, Cy, 5-FU	72%	7

Cy = Cyclophosphamide	Vcr = Vincristine
Mtx = Methotrexate	Pred = Prednisone
5-FU = 5-Fluorouracil	Adria = Adriamycin

Table 5–3.

A 5-drug Combination Chemotherapy Regimen for Metastatic Breast Cancer

Drug	Dose	Route	Treatment schedule
Cyclophosphamide	50–100 mg	Orally	Daily for duration of treatment.
Prednisone	50 mg	Orally	Daily for first three weeks.
	30 mg	Orally	Daily for next two weeks.
	10 mg	Orally	Daily for next one week and then discontinue.
Methotrexate	25 mg	I.V.	Every 7 days × 6 doses
5-Fluorouracil	500 mg	I.V.	and then every 14 days
Vincristine	1.0 mg	I.V.	for duration of treatment.

apeutic regimen, chemotherapy is maintained until relapse occurs. Cessation of chemotherapy often results in rapid relapse and thus maintenance chemotherapy is recommended. The mean duration of chemotherapy-induced remissions has been eight to 10 months.

Combination chemotherapy clearly represents a significant advance in the management of metastatic breast cancer. In addition to a high overall response, multidrug therapy results in significantly more complete responses than single-agent therapy. The chemotherapy is generally administered in the outpatient department, so as to minimize time spent away from work and family. However, the toxicity of combination chemotherapy should not be underestimated. The non-life-threatening side effects can include alopecia, nausea, vomiting, mucositis, cystitis. Bone marrow depression is a more serious toxicity which is caused by virtually all the agents except vincristine. Vincristine does result in neurologic toxicity, which can be particularly disabling in elderly patients. Adriamycin results in a dose-related cardiac toxicity, so at the present time the total dose of Adriamycin is limited to 500 to 550 mgm/square meter.

Extensive effort continues in the development of more effective single agents and combinations of drugs for treatment of metastatic breast cancer. However, combination chemotherapy may perhaps be used to greater advantage earlier in the course, i.e., as an adjuvant to surgery in patients who are at a great risk to develop metastatic cancer (19). The encouraging results in adjuvant chemotherapy are described in Chapter 4.

Treatment—Specific Plans

One of the major challenges in the management of metastatic breast cancer is the design of a treatment plan that utilizes the available therapeutic modalities in an optimal sequence. Specific treatment plans for premenopausal and postmenopausal women will be outlined in this section. It must be emphasized that these recommendations represent only one of several alternative approaches to the management of metastatic breast cancer.

In the treatment-flow plans described in the following pages, estrogen receptor assays are used to select patients for hormonal therapy. Estrogen receptor assays certainly appear to be clinically helpful and are now commercially available. However, further investigations into basic biologic and clinical aspects of steroid receptors are necessary before the importance of these receptor assays in the selection of therapeutic modalities can be determined.

Premenopausal Patients. It is unusual to detect an isolated asymptomatic metastasis in a premenopausal woman. If only one asymptomatic metastatic lesion is found on the initial clinical assessment, two or three symptomatic metastases are usually detected within several months. The majority of premenopausal women with recurrent disease are thus candidates for systemic therapy.

Decisions regarding the initial course of systemic therapy should be partly based on the assay of estrogen receptors in the primary tumor and/or metastatic lesion. Those patients with positive estrogen receptor assays are treated initially with castration. An overall response rate of greater than 50 percent can be anticipated.

A significant number of patients will be encountered who have not had the primary tumor analyzed for estrogen receptors and who have metastatic disease which is inaccessible to biopsy. In most of these cases, castration is also the initial therapy of choice, but a response rate of only 30 percent can be predicted without knowledge of estrogen receptors.

Premenopausal women with tumors which contain no estrogen receptors are not candidates for castration, because there is less than a 5 percent chance of response to this ablative procedure in this subgroup of patients. Combination chemotherapy is the initial therapy in these women. Patients with widespread visceral metastases and/or rapidly progressive disease are also candidates for chemotherapy rather than castration, because the extent and pace of their disease demands a rapid antitumor response. The effect of cytotoxic drugs may be apparent within seven days, while the effect of castration can be delayed for many weeks.

Those patients who undergo castration are observed for two to three months for signs of remission. If objective signs of response or stabilization of disease are not noted within this period of time, then the patient should be considered a candidate for chemotherapy. Androgens are reported to be effective in 10 to 20 percent of premenopausal women who did not respond to castration and can be given a trial in those women with indolent tumors which are not producing severe symptoms.

If an objective response to castration is achieved, it is common practice to follow the patient and institute no additional therapy until relapse occurs. Investigational trials are underway to evaluate the effect of oophorectomy with and without added combination chemotherapy on the duration of tumor response and survival in premenopausal patients with metastatic breast cancer (9).

At the time of relapse, the patient who has had a response to castration is a candidate for either a secondary ablative procedure or combination chemotherapy. Hypophysectomy or adrenalectomy is generally selected for those patients who have slowly progressive, local soft tissue or osseous metastases and are in good general medical condition. Those patients who have rapidly progressive disease or visceral involvement receive chemotherapy.

The flow plan for systemic therapy in premenopausal women is outlined in Figure 5-1.

Postmenopausal Patients. The clinical management of postmenopausal women with recurrent breast cancer generally requires more individualization than the management of the premenopausal patient. Prompt and vigorous therapy in premenopausal women is indicated, because these women often have rapidly progressive disease associated with increasingly severe symptoms. In contrast, postmenopausal women will frequently present with clinical and/or radiographic evidence of an isolated metastasis and no symptoms.

Local recurrence on the chest wall or in the axillary or supraclavicular lymph nodes not infrequently appears in older women many years after the primary tumor has been removed. Local treatment is indicated in these patients, even though the lesion may not be producing symptoms, particularly if there is no other evidence of recurrence after the clinical assessment has been completed. Recurrences on the chest wall can usually be excised. If surgical excision is not feasible, irradiation is another effective means of destroying the tumor. If the axillary or supraclavicular lymph nodes are mobile, surgical excision is the preferred method of therapy. Fixed or matted lymph nodes are biopsied to confirm the diagnosis and treated by

Fig. 5-1. Systemic therapy of recurrent or metastatic disease in premenopausal women.

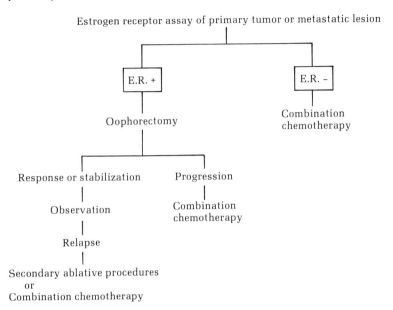

Estrogen receptor assay of primary tumor or metastatic lesion

E.R. +

E.R. -

Oophorectomy

Combination
chemotherapy

Response or stabilization

Progression

Observation

Combination
chemotherapy

Relapse

Secondary ablative procedures
or
Combination chemotherapy

irradiation. Hopefully, irradiation has not been employed as a prophylactic measure following the initial mastectomy. If postoperative irradiation was employed as an adjuvant to primary therapy, the details of the prior irradiation as to dose and fields of irradiation should be reviewed. Additional therapy may be feasible, depending upon the site of recurrence, the previous fields of irradiation, and the type and dose of irradiation employed.

The postmenopausal woman with an isolated bone metastasis which is causing significant pain can be effectively palliated by irradiation. Whether systemic therapy such as estrogens should be administered depends upon the results of the clinical assessment. In the presence of no other evidence of metastases and a long disease-free interval, irradiation alone is preferable. Estrogens are administered in conjunction with irradiation to a patient with a short disease-free interval and other asymptomatic metastases. The presence or absence of estrogen receptors in the cytoplasm of the tumor further delineates the indication for estrogens. Tumors with significant levels of estrogen-binding protein are more apt to respond to estrogens than tumors which contain no estrogen-binding protein in their cytoplasm.

The patient with evidence of two or three sites of recurrence and multiple symptoms is started on estrogens if the tumor cells contain estrogen-binding protein. Patients who have not had their tumor analyzed for estrogen receptors are candidates for estrogen therapy, but a response rate of only 30 percent can be predicted without knowledge of the estrogen-binding protein. In the absence of estrogen-binding protein in the tumor cells and/or in the face of disease which is rapidly progressive or widespread in visceral organs, it is preferable to begin chemotherapy rather than estrogens. Tumors without estrogen-binding protein generally do not respond to any type of hormonal manipulation.

If estrogens are administered, they are continued for at least eight weeks for adequate evaluation of a clinical response. The majority of patients who are going to respond will show some evidence of response within eight weeks. If progression of the disease is noted the drug is discontinued and combination chemotherapy is initiated.

Those patients who have achieved a response are maintained on estrogens until relapse occurs. When estrogens are discontinued at the time of relapse, transient regression of the tumor may occur as a response to estrogen withdrawal in 10 percent of patients. The estrogen responder who has relapsed is then a candidate for androgen therapy, secondary ablative procedures, or combination chemotherapy. As in the premenopausal patient, the choice between hormonal therapy and combination chemotherapy is largely based on the distribution of the metastatic disease, the pace of the cancer, and the general medical status of the patient. The flow plan for systemic treatment of postmenopausal women is outlined in Figure 5-2.

Patients in Immediate Postmenopausal Years. Patients who are between one and four years postmenopausal have generally not been good responders to endocrine therapy. In this age group, combination chemotherapy is generally recommended as the initial form of systemic therapy. The availability of steroid receptor assays may aid in the selection of patients for endocrine therapy in the immediate postmenopausal years. At the current time, however, endocrine therapy should be reserved for patients in this age group who have indolent soft tissue or osseous metastases.

Common Problems Encountered in Both Premenopausal and Postmenopausal Patients

In all patients with recurrent or metastatic breast cancer, whether they are premenopausal, menopausal or postmenopausal, a number

Fig. 5-2. Systemic therapy of recurrent or metastatic disease in postmenopausal women.

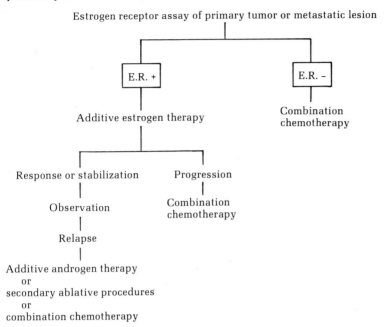

Estrogen receptor assay of primary tumor or metastatic lesion

E.R. +

E.R. –

Additive estrogen therapy

Combination chemotherapy

Response or stabilization

Progression

Observation

Combination chemotherapy

Relapse

Additive androgen therapy
    or
secondary ablative procedures
    or
combination chemotherapy

of complications arise which are managed in a similar fashion. Although an infinite number of complications can be encountered, certain complications are common enough to warrant individual discussion.

Management of the Primary Breast Tumor in Patients Who on Initial Evaluation Have Evidence of Distant Metastases. Although subsequent therapy differs according to the menopausal status of the patient, the principles of management of the primary breast cancer in a patient who on initial examination has evidence of distant metastases are similar in both groups. If the primary lesion is small and there is no evidence of skin edema or ulceration, no specific therapy is directed to the primary tumor and the patient is treated with whatever systemic therapy is indicated. However, a primary tumor which has ulcerated the skin causes a good deal of pain and discomfort and also produces a foul odor. This type of lesion is best managed by simple mastectomy if the tumor is not fixed to the chest wall and primary skin closure can be obtained. In the presence of extensive skin involvement, irradiation will usually shrink the tumor and decrease the amount of skin ulceration. In some instances, however, the ulceration persists in spite of the irradiation and healing is dependent upon the effects of systemic therapy.

Management of a Pleural Effusion. A significant pleural effusion causing chest pain and shortness of breath secondary to displacement and collapse of the adjacent lung parenchyma is frequently encountered in patients with metastatic breast cancer. The effusion, which can be either serous or grossly bloody, is caused by the seeding of malignant cells on the visceral and/or parietal surfaces. The effusions are initially aspirated and material obtained for routine bacterial, fungal, and mycobacterial cultures. Cytologic smears of the fluid are examined to confirm the diagnosis of metastatic breast cancer.

Pleural fluid reaccumulation can often be controlled by systemic antitumor therapy and/or periodic thoracentesis. If the fluid reaccumulates within several days or a week, further procedures are necessary. The aim of all procedures is to obliterate the pleural space by creating a symphysis between the visceral and parietal pleura. Three basic methods are available: (1) insertion of a chest tube into the pleural space and the application of suction to the water-sealed drainage bottle; (2) insertion of a chest tube and the instillation of cytotoxic drug prior to applying suction to the water-sealed drainage bottle; (3) thoracotomy and decortication of the visceral and parietal pleura. The first procedure involves inserting a rubber rather than a Silastic catheter into the pleural space. The rubber tube probably induces more of an inflammatory response than a Silastic catheter and therefore more chance of a pleural symphysis. If the rubber tube fails to produce a pleural symphysis and the pleural effusion recurs, a Silastic tube is inserted and the effusion drained. Nitrogen mustard in a dosage of 0.2 mg per kilogram of body weight dissolved in 200 cc of saline is then instilled into the pleural space and the chest tube is clamped. The patient changes positions frequently for thirty minutes and the clamp is removed from the tube and suction applied to the water-sealed bottle for twenty-four hours. The Silastic tube is removed twenty-four hours later. The nitrogen mustard does gain access to the systemic circulation and can cause gastrointestinal and bone marrow toxicity. If the pleural effusion recurs, the entire procedure is repeated in two weeks, provided that the white blood cell count is within normal limits. These procedures, which should be accomplished in a sequential fashion, will prevent further accumulation of pleural fluid in approximately 75 percent of the patients. A few patients are candidates for thoracotomy and decortication. These patients should be in relatively good condition, with a life expectancy of at least one year. Decortication should not be considered in any patient whose lung does not fully re-expand after aspiration of the pleural fluid. If all of these criteria are present, and if all other methods of controlling the pleural effusion have failed, a thoracotomy is performed and the visceral and the parietal pleural excised.

Metastases to the Central Nervous System.   Metastatic lesions in the cerebral hemispheres produce headache, seizures, motor and sensory defects, visual defects, and personality changes. Lesions in the posterior fossa produce headaches, gait disturbances, and vertigo. The presence of metastatic disease in the central nervous system can be confirmed by a brain scan, computerized axial tomography, or arteriogram. The patient with a solitary brain metastasis can at times be effectively palliated by surgical excision of the metastatic lesion. This type of procedure should only be undertaken if the metastasis is detected at least several years after the primary therapy and no other evidence of metastases are detected. In the presence of multiple lesions, which are far more common than solitary metastases, and/or diffuse systemic metastases, the symptoms of brain metastases can be palliated by reducing cerebral edema with dexamethasone and treating the entire brain with irradiation.

Spinal Cord Compression.   Paraplegia as a result of spinal cord compression secondary to collapse of vertebral bodies or extradural masses can be prevented in the majority of patients. In the initial clinical assessment and during any subsequent follow-up visits it is important to try to detect clinical findings indicative of vertebral or epidural metastases. Back pain without other neurologic signs or symptoms may be the first clue to cord compression. Radicular pain, weakness, paresthesias, gait disturbances, bowel or bladder dysfunction, and focal neurologic signs can be later findings of cord compression. Myelography is indicated if cord compression is suspected. If the myelogram reveals a small extradural defect, the patient is fitted with a brace and irradiated. If a block in the spinal canal is demonstrated, an immediate laminectomy is performed and the patient is given postoperative irradiation to eradicate the remaining tumor. Immediate laminectomy is also indicated in those patients who suddenly develop paraplegia. Following decompression of the spinal cord, the tumor is treated by irradiation. Steroids are useful in reducing edema secondary to the tumor or the radiation therapy.

Pathologic Fractures. Seventy-five percent of the patients who die with metastic breast cancer have evidence of bone metastases at autopsy, both osteolytic and osteoblastic lesions. Osteoblastic lesions usually do not cause a subsequent fracture, but osteolytic lesions coalesce and frequently cause a pathologic fracture. There are a significant number of patients with pelvic or proximal femoral involvement. Pathologic fractures of either hip or the femur cause severe pain and loss of function. Palliative measures are designed to relieve pain, restore function, and simplify the patient's care. Although these lesions will respond to irradiation, such treatment is time-consuming and the patient is unable to walk until healing has occurred. An alternative method which appears promising is immediate operation and curettement of the metastatic tumor within the bone. The bone is then stabilized with either a Jewett nail in the hip or an intramedullary nail in the femur. These metal prostheses are fixed in place with methylmethacrilate. Irradiation is begun postoperatively to destroy residual foci of tumor. With continued improvement in orthopedic techniques, consideration should be given to prophylactic surgery for selected patients with lesions in weight-bearing bones that are likely to result in pathologic fracture.

Hypercalcemia. Acute elevation of the serum calcium generally occurs as the result of widespread bony metastases, or can be induced by estrogen or androgen therapy. Hypercalcemia can cause a variety of distressing symptoms such as nausea, vomiting, constipation, polyuria and polydipsia, stupor, and aberrant behavior. The serum calcium may return to normal with vigorous hydration and increased activity. If the serum calcium does not return to normal, mithramycin in a dosage of 25 micrograms per kilogram given intravenously will usually lower the serum calcium within two days. These patients also are placed on a low calcium diet and also oral phosphate (Fleet's phosphosoda 2 teaspoons every four hours).

The Palliation of Severe Pain. The palliation of pain which is not controlled by analgesics is one of the most challenging problems a physician encounters in the management of patients with recurrent breast carcinoma. As previously noted, pain can occur from a variety of causes, but severe constant pain is frequently due to bony metastases. Although a number of these patients initially respond to additive or ablative hormonal therapy or cytotoxic drugs, a significant number of patients do not respond, and almost all patients will eventually relapse after an initial response to these palliative measures. The indications for some type of pain-relief procedure are based on the patient's life expectancy, the location of the metastatic lesion, and the presence or absence of associated neurologic deficits. If the patient is expected to survive for at least several months, a percutaneous cordotomy is indicated. If the pain is below the costal margin a thoracic cordotomy can be performed; if the pain is above this level, a cervical cordotomy is necessary. The cervical procedure can be combined with avulsion of the cervical nerve roots to relieve pain in the neck. Cordotomy often relieves pain from metastatic breast cancer. If a bilateral procedure is necessary, it is associated with a significant incidence of bladder incontinence, dysesthesia and hemiparesis. A cervical cordotomy can also be associated with sleep-induced apnea.

Within the past five years, there has been increasing interest in the development of procedures which will relieve pain but not cause loss of neurologic function. The use of afferent nerve stimulators has been extensively investigated by Long (42) and others. Afferent stimulators utilizing electricity for their input have effectively relieved pain when applied to cutaneous nerves, and these stimulators have also been implanted in peripheral nerves and in the spinal cord. This type of work is still under clinical investigation and firm conclusions cannot be made at the present time. A number of patients with metastatic breast cancer may be relieved of their pain by these techniques, which do not cause the morbidity and mortality which is associated with either open or percutaneous cordotomy.

It is also worth noting recent reports that levodopa (L-Dopa) can relieve bone pain in patients with bone metastases due to breast cancer (46, 47). The mechanism of levodopa's action is not known, although suppression of prolactin was originally suspected. Tolis has pointed out that the relief of bone pain may not be associated with objective improvement of the breast cancer, and therefore the absence of pain may be deceptive to both patient and physician (52).

Psychologic Support for the Patient and Family. Breast cancer is, in many ways, a chronic illness in which the patient can experience multiple remissions and relapses. An effective treatment program not only requires technical expertise in surgery, radiation therapy, and drug therapy but also a concerned and compassionate staff of physicians and nurses who can help the patient cope psychologically with the multiple problems arising from her illness. The medical staff must be sufficiently flexible to provide optimism and encouragement during periods of recovery and rehabilitation and yet help the patient accept the realities of her disease and the limitations of therapy.

Formal psychiatric consultation is probably not necessary for the majority of patients with breast cancer, and, in fact, is not feasible for this large number of patients. However, a self-administered psychologic testing instrument that could help to identify patients who are in need of increased psychological support and/or formal psychiatric consultation would be a valuable addition to the diagnostic evaluation and follow-up of patients with breast cancer. The SCL-90 is a screening instrument that has been developed in the Department of Psychiatry at The Johns Hopkins Hospital and has been found to be quite useful in detecting psychologic symptomatology in psychiatric outpatients and patients with a variety of medical illnesses. The initial trials with the SCL-90 in patients with hematologic malignancies and solid tumors have been encouraging (1, 15). More detailed studies of the SCL-90 in patients with primary and metastatic breast cancer are currently under way.

Virtually all patients with metastatic breast cancer will eventually become refractory to antitumor therapy. At this point in the illness, increasing attention must be directed at psychologic support of the patient and her family. Although most patients die in the hospital, it is becoming more common for families to request that the patient spend as much time as possible at home during the terminal phase of the illness. Adequate home care can often be arranged, with the help of the visiting nurses and social service agencies.

Pain and apprehension are two major problems of the dying patient. These symptoms can often be partly relieved by the combination of a narcotic and a phenothiazine. Percodan and chlorpromazine constitute a particularly effective combination. There has been a great deal of interest in the use of Elavil and Prolixin as an analgesic regimen. Our results have been somewhat discouraging with these drugs, although the antidepressant effects of Elavil can be most helpful.

During the course of the illness, and particularly during the terminal stages, a great deal of attention and support is provided to the patient and her family. It is important to recognize that many families can benefit from continuing support and counseling (particularly from nurses and social workers) following the death of their relative.

References

1. Abeloff, M. D., and Derogatis, L. 1975. Psychiatric symptomatology in oncology patients: A quantitative approach. *Proc. Am. Soc. Clin. Oncol.* 16:235.
2. Ansfield, F. J., Ramirez, G., Machman, S., et al. 1969. A ten-year study of 5-fluorouracil in disseminated breast cancer with clinical results and survival times. *Cancer Research* 29:1062.
3. Ansfield, F. J., Davis, H. L., Ellerby, R. A., and Ramirez, G. 1974. A clinical trial of megestrol acetate in advanced breast cancer. *Cancer* 33:907.
4. Baker, L. H., Vaughn, C. B., Al-Sarraf, M., et al. 1974. Evaluation of combination vs. sequential cytotoxic chemotherapy in the treatment of advanced breast cancer. *Cancer* 33:513.
5. Beatson, G. T., 1896. On the treatment of inoperable cases of carcinoma of the mamma: Suggestions for a new method of treatment with illustrative cases. *Lancet* 2:104.
6. Blum, R. H., and Carter, S. K. 1974. Adriamycin—a new anticancer drug with significant clinical activity. *Ann. Intern. Med.* 80:249.
7. Blumenschein, G. R., Cardenas, J. O., Freireich, E. J., and Gottlieb, J. A. 1974. FAC chemotherapy for breast cancer. *Proc. Am. Soc. Clin. Oncol.* 15:193. (Abstr.).
8. Carter, S. K. 1972. Single and combination nonhormonal chemotherapy in breast cancer. *Cancer* 30:1543.
9. Carter, S. K. 1974. The chemical therapy of breast cancer. *Seminars in Oncology* 1:131.
10. Conway, L. W., and Collins, W. F. 1969. Results of transphenoidal cryohypophysectomy for carcinoma of the breast. *New Engl. J. Med.* 281:1.
11. Cooper, R. J. 1969. Combination chemotherapy in hormone resistant breast cancer. *Proc. Am. Assoc. Cancer Res.* 10:15. (Abstr.).
12. Cooperative Breast Cancer Group. 1961. Progress report—results of studies by the Cooperative Breast Cancer Group—1956-60. *Cancer Chemother. Rep.* 11:130.
13. Council on Drugs, Subcommittee on Breast and Genital Cancer, Committee on Research, AMA. 1960. Androgens and estrogens in the treatment of disseminated mammary carcinoma—retrospective study of 944 patients. *JAMA* 172:1271.
14. Costanza, M. E., Saroj, D., Nathanson, L., et al. 1974. Carcinoembryonic antigen. Report of a screening study. *Cancer* 33:583.
15. Craig, T. J., and Abeloff, M. D. 1974. Psychiatric symptomatology among hospitalized oncology patients. *Am. J. Psych.* 131:1321.
16. DeLena, M., Brembella, C., Morabeto, A., and Bonadonna, G. 1975. Adriamycin plus vincristine compared to and conbined with cyclophosphamide, methotrexate, and 5-fluorouracil for advanced breast cancer. *Cancer* 35:1108.
17. DeVita, V. T., Jr., Serpick, A. A., and Carbone, P. P. 1970. Combination chemotherapy in the treatment of advanced Hodgkin's disease. *Ann. Intern. Med.* 73:881.
18. Fisher, B. 1968. Surgical adjuvant chemotherapy in cancer of the breast. *Ann. Surg.* 168:337.
19. Fisher, B. F., Carbone, P., Economou, S. G., et al. 1975. L-phenylalanine mustard (L-PAM) in the management of primary breast cancer. *New Engl. J. Med.* 292:117.
20. Folca, P. J., Gascock. R. F., Irvine, W. T. 1961. Studies with tritium-labeled hexoestrol in advanced breast cancer. *Lancet* 2:796.
21. Fracchia, A. A., Randall, H. T., Farrow, J. H. 1967. The results of adrenalectomy in advanced breast cancer in 500 consecutive patients. *Surg. Gynec. Obstet.* 125:747.
22. Fracchia, A. A., Farrow, J. H., Miller, T. R., et al. 1971. Hypophysectomy as compared to adrenalectomy for advanced breast cancer. *Surg. Gynec. Obstet.* 133:241.

23. Freireich, E. J., Karon, M., and Frei, E., III. 1964. Quadruple combination therapy (VAMP) for acute lymphocytic leukemia of childhood. *Proc. Am. Assoc. Cancer Res.* 5:20 (Abstr.).

24. Gold, P., and Freedman, S. O. 1965. Demonstration of tumor-specific antigens in human colonic carcinomata by immunological and absorption techniques. *J. Exp. Med.* 121:439.

25. Gottlieb, J. G., Bonnet, J. D., Hoogstraten, B., et al. 1973. Superiority of adriamycin over oral nitrosoureas in patients with breast cancer. *Cancer Chemother. Rep.* 57:98.

26. Greenspan, E. 1963. Response of advanced breast cancer to the combination of antimetabolite, methotrexate, and the alkylating agent, thio-TEPA. *J. Mt. Sinai Hospital, N.Y.* 30:246.

27. Greenspan, E. 1966. Combination cytotoxic chemotherapy in advanced disseminated breast cancer. *J. Mt. Sinai Hospital, N.Y.* 33:1.

28. Griffiths, C. T., Hall, T. C., Saba, Z., Barlow, J. J., and Nevanny, H. B. 1973. Preliminary trail of aminoglutethimide in breast cancer. *Cancer* 32:31.

29. Hoogstraten, B., Owens, A. H., Lenhard, R. E., Jr., et al. 1969. Combination chemotherapy in lymphosarcoma and reticulum cell sarcoma. *Blood* 33:370.

30. Horwitz, K. B., McGuire, W. L., Pearson, O. H., and Segaloff, A. 1975. Predicting response to endocrine therapy in human breast cancer: A hypothesis. *Science* 189:726.

31. Jensen, E. V., Block, G. E., Smith, S., Kyser, K., and Desombre, E. R. 1971. Estrogen receptors and breast cancer response to adrenalectomy. Prediction of response in cancer therapy. *Natl. Cancer Inst. Monogr.* 34:55.

32. Jones, S. E., Durie, B. G. M., and Salmon, S. E. 1975. Combination chemotherapy with adriamycin and cyclophosphamide for advanced breast cancer. *Cancer* 36:90.

33. Kennedy, B. J., Theologides, A., Fortuny, I., Foley, J., and Brown, J. 1964. Diethylstilbesterol and testosterone propionate therapy in advanced breast cancer. *Cancer Chemother. Rep.* 41:11.

34. Kennedy, B. J., and Fortuny, I. E. 1964. Therapeutic castration in the treatment of advanced breast cancer. *Cancer* 17:1197.

35. Kennedy, B. J., Mielke, P. W., Fortuny, I. E. 1964. Therapeutic castration versus prophylactic castration in breast cancer. *Surg. Gynec. Obstet.* 118:524.

36. Kennedy, B. J. 1974. Hormonal therapies in breast cancer. *Seminars in Oncology* 1:119.

37. Kelly, R. M. 1971. Hormonal chemotherapy in breast cancer. *Cancer* 28:1686.

38. Korenman, S. G., Dukes, D. 1970. Specific estrogen binding by the cytoplasm of human breast cancer. *J. Clin. Endocrin.* 30:639.

39. Lee, J. M., Abeloff, M. D., Lenhard, R. E., and Baker, R. R. 1974. An evaluation of five drug combination chemotherapy in the management of recurrent carcinoma of the breast. *Surg. Gynec. Obstet.* 138:77.

40. Lenhard, R. E., Jr. 1971. Clinical case records in chemotherapy: The management of hypercalcemia complicating cancer. *Cancer Chemother. Rep.* 55:509.

41. Lipton, A., and Santen, R. J. 1974. Medical adrenalectomy using aminoglutethemide and dexamethasone in advanced breast cancer. *Cancer* 33:503.

42. Long, D. M. 1974. External electrical stimulation as a treatment for pain. *Minn. Med.* 57:195.

43. MacDonald, I. 1962. Endrocrine ablation in disseminated mammary cancer. *Surg. Gynec. Obstet.* 115:215.

44. McGuire, W. L. 1973. Estrogen receptors in human breast cancer. *J. Clin. Invest.* 52:73.

45. McGuire, W. L., Pearson, O. H., Segaloff, A. 1975. *Estrogen receptors in human breast cancer*, W. L. McGuire, P. P. Carbone, E. P. Vollmer, eds. New York: Raven.

46. Minton, J. P. 1974. The response of breast cancer patients with bone pain to L-dopa. *Cancer* 33:358.
47. Nixon, D. W. 1975. Use of L-dopa to relieve pain from bone metastases. *New Engl. J. Med.* 292:647.
48. Steward, A. M., Nixon, D., Zamcheck, N., and Aisenberg, A. 1974. Carcinoembryonic antigens in breast cancer patients: Serum levels and disease progress. *Cancer* 33:1252.
49. Taft, D., and Gorski, J. 1966. A receptor for estrogen. Isolation from rat uterus and preliminary characterization. *Proc. Natl. Acad. Sci. USA*, 55:1574.
50. Taylor, S. G., III, Canellos, G. P., Band, P., et al. 1974. Combination chemotherapy for advanced breast cancer: randomized comparison with single drug therapy. *Proc. Am. Soc. Clin. Onc.* 15:175 (Abstr.).
51. Terenius, L., Johannsson, H., Rimsten, A., and Thoren, L. 1974. Malignant and benign mammary disease estrogen binding in relation to clinical data. *Cancer* 33:1364.
52. Tolis, G. J. 1975. L-dopa for pain from bone metastases. *New Engl. J. Med.* 292:1352.
53. Tormey, D. C., Waalkes, T. P., Ahmann, D., et al. 1975. Biologic markers in breast carcinoma. I. Incidence of abnormalities of CEA, HCG, three polyamines, and three minor nucleosides. *Cancer* 35:1095.
54. Wilson, R. R., Piro, A. J., Aliapoulios, M. A., and Moore, F. A. 1971. Treatment of metastatic breast cancer with a combination of adrenalectomy and 5-fluorouracil. *Cancer* 28:962.
55. Wittliff, J. L. 1974. Specific receptors of the steroid hormones in breast cancer. *Seminars in Oncology* 1:109.

CONTRIBUTORS

Martin D. Abeloff, M.D. Assistant Professor of Oncology and Instructor of Medicine, The Johns Hopkins University School of Medicine

R. Robinson Baker, M.D. Professor of Surgery and Oncology, The Johns Hopkins University School of Medicine, and Surgeon-in-Charge, Breast Clinic, The Johns Hopkins Hospital

Darryl Carter, M.D. Associate Professor of Pathology and Oncology, The Johns Hopkins University School of Medicine

Joseph C. Eggleston, M.D. Associate Professor of Pathology and Oncology, The Johns Hopkins University School of Medicine

Atsuko Heshiki, M.D. Assistant Professor of Radiology, The Johns Hopkins University School of Medicine

Morton L. Levin, M.D., Dr.P.H. Professor of Epidemiology, The Johns Hopkins University School of Hygiene

Floyd Osterman, Jr., M.D. Fellow in Radiology, The Johns Hopkins University School of Medicine

David B. Thomas, M.D., Dr.P.H. Associate Professor of Epidemiology, The Johns Hopkins University School of Hygiene

AUTHOR INDEX

SUBJECT INDEX

Library of Congress Cataloging in Publication Data

Main entry under title:
Current trends in the management of breast cancer.

  Includes bibliographical references.
  1: Breast—Cancer. I. Baker, Ralph Robinson, 1928-
[DNLM: 1. Breast neoplasms. WP870 C976]

RC280.B8C78   616.9'94'49   76-49094
ISBN 0-8018-1858-3